The Diet-Free Diet Book

Other books by Janet Hunt

A Vegetarian in the Family
The Holistic Cook
Natural Sweets
Pasta Dishes
Pizzas and Pancakes
Quiches and Flans
The Raw Food Way to Health
Simple and Speedy Wholefood Cookery
Vegetarian Snacks and Starters
365 plus 1 Vegetarian Main Meals
The Wholefood Lunch Box
The Wholefood Sweets Book
Italian Dishes
The Compassionate Gourmet

all the above published by Thorsons

The Complete Vegetarian Cookbook

published by Hamlyn

The Caring Cook

published by The Vegan Society

The Diet-Free Diet Book

Janet Hunt

Illustrations by
Viv Quillin

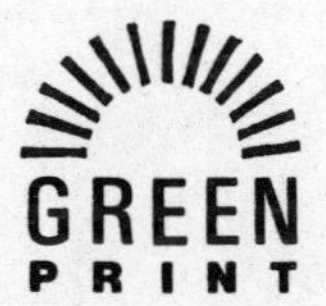

First published in 1990 by
Green Print
an imprint of The Merlin Press
10 Malden Road, London NW5 3HR

ISBN 1 85425 042 6

1 2 3 4 5 6 7 8 9 10 :: 99 98 97 96 95 94 93 92 91 90

Phototypeset by Computerset Phototypesetting Ltd., Harmondsworth

Printed in England by Biddles Ltd., Guildford, Surrey on recycled paper

Contents

Unless otherwise specified, the word *diet* is used to mean a strict regime followed in order to lose weight.

Introduction

Although the facts given on the following pages have been gleaned from and/or checked with nutritionalists, dieticians, doctors and practitioners in natural medicine – all of whom I thank – this is in no way claiming to be a medical book. My aim in writing it is to tell those many people (both female and male, all shapes and sizes) who are tired of trying to change themselves by dieting, that health and happiness *are* possible. That you can have a body of which you are proud, *and* enjoy eating real food, *and* feel fit and full of energy.

How?

Firstly throw out all the diet books, the scales, the saccharin, the calorie counter and whatever other weapons you've acquired to help you fight the war against yourself.

Secondly – just for a while – forget completely about how you look. This might not come easily if you're in the habit of worrying about what the rest of the world thinks of you, but try. Find a quiet place where you can concentrate without interruption, maybe for a hour each evening. Better still, take a few days off – a weekend would be ideal. Go right away. Or lock the front door, take the telephone off the hook, disconnect the bell. Wear what you feel most comfortable in, relax, switch off about everything except this book.

Thirdly, start reading.

This isn't, however, just a book to be read. To get maximum benefit from it, you'll need to do a little work. At the start of each chapter you'll find a quiz. These have been carefully devised to help you find out more about your attitude to yourself, to food, to weight, to your whole way of life. Only by really understanding these things will you be able to start working towards your ideal you! There are no right or wrong answers, no scores to be achieved. Simply answer each question as honestly as you can, thinking carefully before you do so. Some are very simple and their reasons for being there quite obvious, but others may require that you dig deep into your subconscious. Write down your answers if you like. The chapter following each quiz will touch on the points raised, showing how to use your answers as stepping stones to success.

The last section of the book is devoted to more practical matters. It shows you how to put into practice everything you've learnt, how to stop dieting once and for all and start living.

Enjoy it – and the rest of your life.

Note: Though this approach to weight problems and health will undoubtedly benefit everyone, it is aimed principally at those who consider themselves to be of average build. Anyone who is genuinely convinced that they are severely over- or underweight would be wise to also seek professional help.

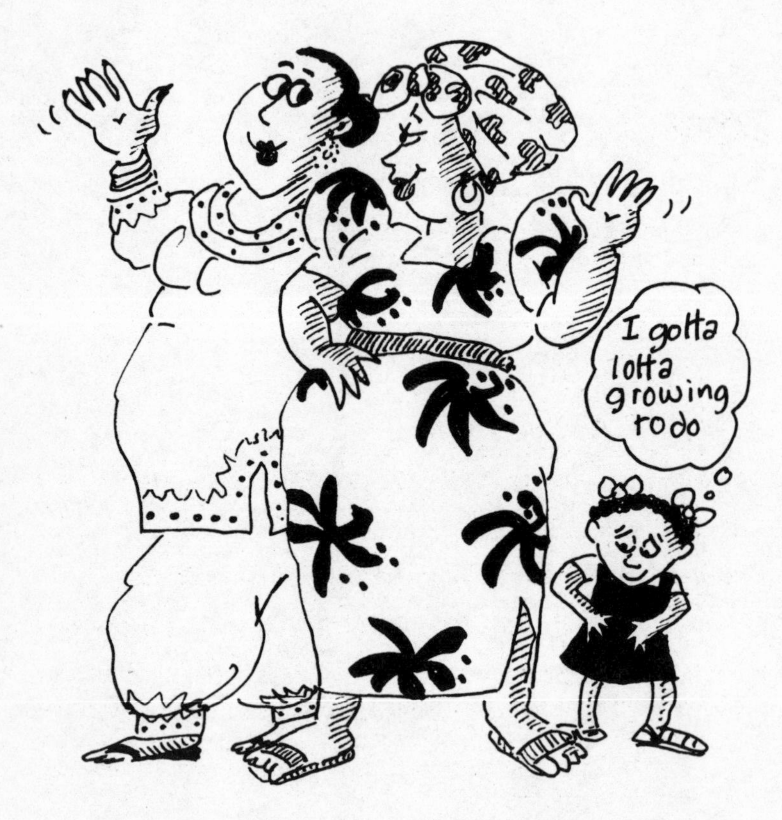

In many parts of the world, a well rounded woman will dress imaginatively

1 *T*his dieting business

QUIZ

1 Are you on a diet right now?
2 Have you ever dieted before?
3 If so, how many times?
  a) twice?
  b) five times?
  c) ten times?
  d) more?
4 What made you give up?
5 Have you ever fasted?
6 Have you ever binged to the point where you felt ill?
7 When dieting, do you find you cannot stop thinking about food?
8 Does dieting in any way affect your day-to-day life
  a) socially?
  b) at work?
  c) with your family?
9 Why do you feel you need to lose weight anyway? Is it because
  a) you are larger than the models you admire in magazines?
  b) you are heavier than your friends?
  c) clothes in shops don't seem to fit you?
10 If trying to gain weight, have you ever found yourself physically revolted at the thought of eating?

The fashion for dieting

Chances are that if you're reading this it's because you're unhappy about your weight. You might feel you're too thin and long to gain a few pounds. It's more likely though that excess weight is your problem; whatever friends and family might say about you being 'just right', you know they're trying to be nice and deep down inside you still feel you're fat and ugly! You have only to flick through a fashion magazine to have your doubts confirmed. Maybe you've tried to do something about changing your shape and failed. Or achieved your aim and then gradually, without even noticing, reverted to eating the way you used to, and put back the pounds you worked so hard to lose.

Dieting may well have become an intrinsic part of your life, colouring everything you do. Eating out with friends, going on holiday, buying new clothes. It's always there, taking over from the church with its insistence that you behave yourself, practise self-denial – and if you do give in to temptation, weak and sinful as you are, making sure you not only feel guilty about it afterwards, but are punished. Two days on salad and cottage cheese only, says your diet sheet. Better still, crispbread and water.

It it's any consolation, you're not alone. Especially if you're female. Nowadays dieting seems to be seen by many in the western world as a girl's initiation into womanhood. At school it's whispered about; something older sisters and mothers might do. How grown up to be able to say those magic words: I'm on a diet.

This hasn't always been so. Just a few centuries ago, a young man seeking a wife would have had as his ideal a girl with a well-rounded figure, full pink cheeks, wide hips. When compared with her skinny friends she'd be likely to work harder, bear stronger children, and would probably live longer too. Not to mention the obvious advantages of cuddling up close to her on cold nights.

Even today there are many societies that prefer their women to be voluptuous, seeing the more feminine shape as not just more beautiful, but as an Earth Mother figure. It has to be admitted that in some of these societies women have yet to assert themselves as equals to men. But in others there is a happy balance of roles which may well be based on an acceptance and appreciation of the differences between the sexes.

The beauty of such women has proved irresistible to great artists through the ages. Titian was one of the first to immortalise it on canvas; in more recent years there were Gauguin's dusky Tahitian maidens, Toulouse-Lautrec's somehow innocent-looking young prostitutes. The paintings of Watteau, Rubens, Renoir, Courbet and Rembrandt are full of naked flesh, softly blushing and extremely sensual.

It was no doubt the sensual quality of the fuller body that so disgusted the nineteenth-century aesthetics. Suddenly everything changed. Women – at least, middle and upper class women – were required to read books and listen to chamber music and look refined whilst doing so. To be shapely and have pink cheeks was coarse. To be interested in food was to behave like a peasant. They ate next to nothing, strapped themselves (with a little help from their buxom maids!) into corsets, took enemas. When they fainted – as they frequently did – it proved their finesse, their fragility.

Though that extreme phase passed with the Victorians, dieting never quite went out of fashion. Then, over the past few decades, it came back in again, and with a vengeance.

Reasons unlimited

Why? Most certainly one reason is rising affluence and the way of life that accompanies it. We not only eat better and more often, but our lives are full of labour-saving devices that take the strain out of housework, shopping, getting from one place to another. All well and good, of course, but the result is that it's very easy to put on an extra few pounds. Our social lives are richer, we travel the world. And we have more free time in which to worry about our weight. Research by Weightwatchers, world leader in the group weight loss market, showed that though triggers for going on a diet can include Christmas, weddings and other special events, it is the prospect of going on holiday that accounts for one third of all diets started.

There are, however, many other reasons given for dieting, some by those who hope to justify themselves, others by professionals who claim to study the phenomena objectively. One is that with today's near equality of the sexes in the world of big business, women also desire to have taut, streamlined bodies, just like their male counterparts. The image is functional, though; the aim to have a unisex body that goes with the short hair cut, the trousers suit and the briefcase, And certainly there *is* an affinity between slimness and maleness, just as the fertility symbols found in other parts of the world, and still used by many primitive societies, are usually of excessively fat women.

Though the women's liberation movement of the sixties and seventies might well have been the starting point for this equality, the originators of it were very different. In an effort to prove women did not have to live up to men's expectations of them, they encouraged their followers to be themselves, to accept and love their bodies whatever size and shape they were, to burn their diet sheets along with their bras. Unfortunately the media then depicted them as overweight hippies, which was undeserved and did little for the image of the movement. Though their cry for equal rights was taken up and has, to a considerable extent, become widely accepted, their theory that women are under no obligation to look like they've just fallen out of a magazine was sadly lost somewhere along the way.

Another reason suggested is tied up with the youth-cult that has such a strong hold in many western societies. A natural part of ageing is for a woman's body to fill out, to soften. In countries such as those of southern Europe, the woman in her middle years is considered to be at her best, both mentally and physically. A ripe plum, full and fragrant rose. In Britain and America, though, it isn't life that begins at forty; it's the menopause. A woman can't change her age, but she can – with enough determination and money – maintain or re-gain the figure of a young girl. It's not unusual these days to see a middle aged women in jeans and trainers with tiny waist, trim hips, the only give-away being a face that just doesn't quite match the rest of her.

Or do women diet so that they can have a feeling of being in control? In a world very much out of control, where the only thing sure is that nothing is sure, and where a woman's place even in the home with her family may no longer exist, dieting may be one positive thing to do. She can set the rules, can actually change the shape of her body. Nobody else can interfere. She is the one in control, the boss.

Severe overweight is dangerous

Some women determine to lose weight for health reasons, and if they are severly overweight they may be right to do so. The usual way of judging is to calculate anything twenty percent above the amount given on the health insurance charts. For example, if the weight recommended is ten stone, anything above twelve stone might be considered excessive. Statistics show that the severly overweight run an increased risk of developing certain health problems, the most common being heart disease, high blood pressure, diabetes, arthritis, disorders of the gall bladder and thyroid. Conversely, some of these conditions may actually lead to weight gain, and of course this shouldn't be allowed to continue unchecked. However, different recommended weights are given for people who are small, medium and large boned, and if you study them you'll see that they vary considerably, and that even the insurance companies seem to see no great advantage in being as thin as possible. And they should know!

It should be mentioned here that overweight conditions brought about by glandular disorders are a different thing altogether. For many years glands were given as a classic excuse, yet anyone suffering in this way will have many other symptoms too. They may feel tired and lethargic, their thinking fuzzy, they may feel cold much of the time and their hair may become thin. The distribution of any excess weight is also a key to glandular problems: a sufferer may be moon-faced and have body fat, but thin legs. This condition needs to be treated medically, though because it occurs as a result of hormonal malfunctioning, a healthy eating plan can certainly be of benefit as a supplement to drugs.

Probably the saddest reason why women diet – and it may be the most common – is that they are unhappy. They may be lonely, or unsuccessful with their studies or work. They may be getting on in years, or very young and insecure. They may be shy or have pimples or hate their hair. Somewhere along the way an image of the slim woman has built up. She is beautiful, successful, desirable, confident, the life and soul of any party. Becoming slim, therefore, must be the key to happiness. Unfortunately, there is no truth to this. Losing weight guarantees nothing except a looser waistband.

Whatever the reasons though, women do diet. So do many men. It is estimated that almost nine out of ten adults in Britain will have been on at least one diet in their lifetime. Three quarters of them will go on to try as many as five times more, so that their lives will be interspersed at regular intervals with restricted eating regimes. It's official: dieting is a national obsession.

A diet by any other name

No wonder the very word 'diet' has become so very powerful. To sell a magazine, newspaper or book, all you have to do is come up with some new diet. Thus we've had the Grapefruit Diet, the Cottage Cheese Diet, the Junk Food Diet, the Brown Rice Diet, the Champagne Diet, the Lemon and Watercress Diet, the Liquorice All-sorts Diet, the Pritkin Diet, the Scarsdale Diet, the Mayo Diet, the Rotation Diet, the Onion Diet, the Eight Meals a Day Diet, the Low Carbohydrate Diet, the Potato Diet, the Persian Fruit Soup Diet. Some promise you can eat all you want and still lose weight, others insist nothing but a near fast will do. There have been diets for certain areas, like the Hip and Thigh Diet, the Anti-Cellulite Diet. Diets that involve eating everything raw, or boiled, or preceded by a grapefruit, or followed by a spoonful of yogurt.

From American came a scientific diet that read like a chemistry text book – and was about as difficult to understand. The highly popular F-Plan Diet claimed a quicker weight loss on the assumption that much of what you ate would go through you too quickly to be digested! The Cambridge Diet keeps you from starving – just – by allowing you three mini meals supplied in the form of food substitutes, powdered or in bars, that are actually fortified milk and soya products.

In fact, any crash diet will result in rapid weight loss, but this will consist principally *not* of lost fat but of water together with glycogen (which provides an immediately available source of energy) plus lean body tissue. What's more, if a crash diet is continued for any length of time, the body will adjust to such very small meals, becoming super-efficient so that nothing is wasted of this meagre fare. The problems start when the dieter returns to eating relatively normal food; because her metabolism is now so slow she will tend to put on weight despite following a sensible eating plan.

Special diet foods are another way in which manufacturers have latched on to the widespread obsession with losing weight. Many of them, in fact, have little nutritional value, and have as many if not more calories than the conventional equivalents that can be bought for half the price.

Of course, having the willpower to stick to any diet for longer than a day is often the problem. That's where slimming clubs come into the picture. There are a number of chains of them now in Britain alone, all of which follow much the same format. Members pay a fee for which they are entitled to go along to regular meetings and share their problems with other dieters, are praised for any advances they've made, have their resolution recharged for the weeks ahead. The knowledge that any weight gain will be announced out loud to the entire audience – and the anticipation of the shame this will bring – is considered to be a genuine help during times of temptation. Interestingly, ninety percent of the clientele of such clubs are women.

For the more affluent, there are health farms where you can get someone else to supply the willpower for you in the quietly reverential atmosphere – more often than not – of a stately home or country mansion. Echoes of the church again?

With up to some forty percent of American children being overweight, a new idea is Fat Camps to which parents can send their youngsters for the summer, and where they will undoubtedly lose at least a few pounds, probably more – if they stay the course. As in most cases it is the eating habits they have learned at home that account for the children's excess weight, the problem is usually only solved temporarily, but presumably that is enough to allay any guilt the parents might feel.

And if restricting food doesn't do the trick, there are other and more drastic methods to be tried. Hypnotism, either by a practitioner or using a tape or video. Those with a hectic schedule can play a tape whilst they sleep and let the soft, melodious voice work on their subconscious. There are appetite suppressants that contain bulking agents to make you feel full. Amphetamines to take away your appetite, other pills to stimulate the metabolism. Currently under research is a beta adronoceptor antagonist drug that appears to burn off fat; those that have tried it so far say that it made them feel unsteady and shaky, but that it was worth it. People will put up with a lot to lose weight. Some pay to have a surgeon slice off that spare tyre, or wire up their teeth, or give them a gastroplasty, an operation which involves stapling off most of the stomach so they'll feel full on one crispbread.

And yet still, with so many options available, it's a sad fact that seven out of ten who try dieting once go on to become chronic dieters. They might lose a little weight or a lot, stay on their diets for a morning or a year, but eventually the majority of them will re-gain the weight they've lost. Dieting at best is a lost cause. Many times it leads to problems when the dieter becomes tense, tired, even depressed, and is unable to cope. Life at home and work can be adversely affected, relationships strained. Women may also experience physical changes such as irregular periods, with the result that in later years there may be fertility problems.

Eating disorders

At worst dieting can lead to one of the eating disorders about which we hear more and more these days. Compulsive eating that has the victim ransacking every cupboard, eating anything that comes to hand in combinations that, once upon a time, would have revolted her. Usually – and understandably – the compulsive eater also suffers from depression. The next step can be bulimia, when a bout of compulsive eating (or even a normal meal) is followed by the taking of laxatives or induced vomiting. It is at this stage that the dieter is losing control.

Anorexia nervosa may affect the sufferer in much the same way; or it may work in the opposite way, making food seem so repulsive that she cannot bear to eat a thing, longs only to be skinny enough to be able to feel her bones. The important difference is that she eats very little at all. More accurately termed a neurosis, anorexia is most common in teenagers and young women, and is almost as hard for their family to watch as it is to experience. Whilst the anorexic genuinely believes she looks more beautiful with each pound she loses, she may actually become skeletal, so weak she can hardly move, and her inner organs may stop functioning. Though hormonal changes may have something to do with this horrifying illness, psychiatrists suspect links in many cases with mother-figure problems, the girl having a subconscious desire to gain attention maybe, or to compete, or to punish her mother. But whether the causes are physical or psychological, it is an illness that has emerged only in recent years, that is on the increase, and is almost certainly accentuated by the media insistence that women must be slim if they are to be attractive, successful, loved.

Some anorexics can be helped back to good health. Many of them recover but may carry with them the scars for the rest of their lives; for example, they may be unable to have children. A few of them die.

Depressing, hard work, dangerous

So dieting is depressing, hard work, and can also be dangerous. Most of those who diet – at least after the first time – are fully aware of these facts. For whatever reason, they're prepared to have another go. Like a boxer who's been floored they're back on their feet and raring to prove themselves. This time they'll do it, this time they'll show everyone.

Why then do they usually fail? Why is it that so many normal, intelligent people become chronic dieters, trying again and again, forever finding a new diet that is going to be the The One (guaranteed not to fail, it says in the magazine or book)? Where are they going wrong?

Where are *you* going wrong?

One possibility, and consider this carefully, is that maybe you don't need to lose weight. Genetic factors are the strongest influence on your shape, and though you may be able to *adjust* it, your bone structure will obviously remain the same throughout your life. Besides, as in ancient times, the body that is gently rounded may well be at its best: strong, healthy, working with all the efficiency of a well maintained machine. If you feel comfortable in your body, why let a few media people and profit-orientated businessmen dictate that you should be thinner? In an age where everyone is striving to be an individual, to assert their place on this planet, to stand out from the masses, to think for themselves, it is amazing how the desire to have exactly the same size hips as everyone else persists. If your shape is different from your neighbour's, fine. If the clothes you like seem to only come in sizes that don't fit you, why should that automatically mean there's something wrong with you? It is said that half the female population of Britain takes size 16 or over – maybe it's time the manufacturers took in the fact and expanded their ranges instead of insisting you reduce your size.

Even today, in many parts of the world, a well-rounded woman will dress imaginatively, walk with her head held high, proud of her body, confident that she has every right to expect admiration. And because of her attitude, she gets it. It is this obsession with slimness that has so many women in

Britain feeling that, because they are a few pounds over the average, they are somehow inferior and certainly unattractive. You see them everywhere, dressed in black most likely, partly because the slimming magazines insist that black diminishes size, also because in black they can slip along in the shadows, heads down, and not be noticed.

Whatever your weight, if you look and feel good – if *you* are happy with yourself just as you are – forget about dieting.

Reinforcing the failure message

But maybe you are convinced you need to lose some weight, a few pounds anyway. You've tried it before, got close to your goal, and know that if you were just that bit lighter, you'd be satisfied. Your problem is how to get there – and stay there.

You are not alone. Most people who keep going on diets don't have huge amounts of weight to lose, yet still they fail. And though they may start out determined, each failure reinforces the message that dieting is one of the more unpleasant aspects of life that has to be faced, though not necessarily today. They'll definitely start it next Monday. Or in the spring. Or after that party they're so looking forward to.

Maybe a key to this doubt and procrastination is in the words that we have all come to associate with dieting. Think about them.

Willpower. Repression. Discipline. Control. Restraint. Curb. Keep in check. Remove temptation. Sublimate. Sacrifice. Rules. Regime. Restricted. No thank you. Don't tempt me. I'd like to but I'm not allowed. Food itself is described using a whole new vocabulary. It is now naughty, evil, wicked, sinful. Even calorific has become a dirty word (aren't all foods calorific?)

And if you fail – which needn't necessarily mean anything worse than taking an extra potato, or eating a chunk of cheese that wasn't on your list – then more words come to mind. Weak. Unsuccessful. Self-indulgent. Gluttonous. Undisciplined. Shameful. A cheat. A failure. Followed by self-hate, disgust, guilt, punishment.

In fact, in recent years diets have changed from the very strict regimes suggested some time back, to a new easy-going attitude that tries to convince dieters they can have their cake, eat it, *and* lose weight. When looked at closely, however, these diets are still a long list of do's and don'ts. They still demand that you calculate, analyse, pay for your sins. Have a slice of chocolate fudge cake by all means, but only a boiled egg for dinner. Cream in your coffee? Why not, providing you restrict yourself to one cup a week, drink it in the morning so that your body has all day to use up the calories. And only use single cream, of course. You are on a diet, and must never forget it.

What you are doing, in other words, is declaring war on your body.

It is as though your mind and your body were two completely separate beings. Your mind knows best. It has come to a conclusion, and your body – along with all its very natural cravings that are, after all, based on its *needs* – is going to have to submit, give in.

Much the same head-on collision occurs in the less common but equally distressing case of when someone wants to increase their weight. Though there is certainly less media pressure put on the very thin, and statistically they are likely to live considerably longer than those who are very overweight, many of them long to fill out, be more substantial. Men might feel a thin body is not masculine, whilst women crave a softer, more feminine shape. Recent discussions about whether or not sportsmen and women should be able to use anabolic steroids has focused attention on this way of increasing weight, but most doctors are reluctant to give these powerful drugs to their patients without good reason. Side effects such as increased body hair make them undesirable, for women anyway. And those foods known to increase weight most efficiently – namely, sugars and fats – are not only harmful in excess, but can be difficult to consume in large amounts, and may even be impossible to swallow.

And even if they manage to eat more (carbohydrates are probably their best bet), most of those who are underweight have a very fast metabolic rate that burns up food quickly, so even increasing their intake may have little effect.

A mind of its own

Your body, then, may prove to be a powerful opponent. It may have – so to speak – a mind of its own! The trouble is that our need for food is based on a desire to survive. Food nourishes us, provides the materials with which our cells replace themselves, our muscles stay firm, our hearts beat, our blood flows. Food gives us energy to move, to work, to play. Without food we would die, yet by dieting – either to lose or gain weight – we come into conflict with food, and may end up hating or even fearing it. And because our body – making its instinctive feelings known despite what we may tell it – insists that it wants to be fed, we can come in time to hate our bodies.

Needless to say, there are foods and foods. Some are good for our bodies, others bad, and not just as far as putting on weight is concerned. Located at the base of the brain is a mechanism called the hypothalamus. Its function is to tell you when your body needs food, and then – rather like a thermostatic valve – it will also indicate when your body has had enough. Though the hypothalamus works principally on calorie intake and is not concerned with the source of these calories, a finely tuned body will also know exactly which food will provide the specific nutrients it needs. Most of us have sudden and unexpected cravings for a particular food – a chunk of cheese, an apple, a slice of bread. Treat your body right, learn to listen to it, and you'll find that nine times out of ten it will give you sound advice. Young children have an unerring ability to choose not only good but appropriate foods. Unfortunately, today, many of them will have lost this ability before they are more than a few years old, their appetites distorted already by too many sweet and artificially flavoured foods, by well-meaning parents reinforcing the desire for such foods by associating them with treats, birthday parties, days out. This early learning period is vitally important; eating habits accumulated during childhood can stay with us all our lives. The majority of overweight adults are so as a result of eating patterns acquired in those first few formative years.

To correct this is not as difficult as it might seem. But the very first thing to be done is to change your attitude.

Instead of determining to have your own way, to win, resolve to work *with* your body. Whatever weight it is right this minute, however it looks or feels, it is *your* body, a unique body, the only one you have. It's not so bad either, so why not give it a little love and kindness? Trying to change it by battering it into submission may work on a temporary basis, but sooner or later it will rebel. What's more, it will leave you with the feeling that you've failed once again. Working with your body, going slowly, learning to listen to it, to trust it to let you know exactly what it needs and to stop when it's had enough – that is the only way to success. Feed it good wholesome foods and gradually you will find that not only will it adjust to become the weight that best suits it (and be warned, this may not be Twiggy-thin, but in that case you were never meant to be another Twiggy!), but it will also feel fitter, healthier, more alive than it has felt before.

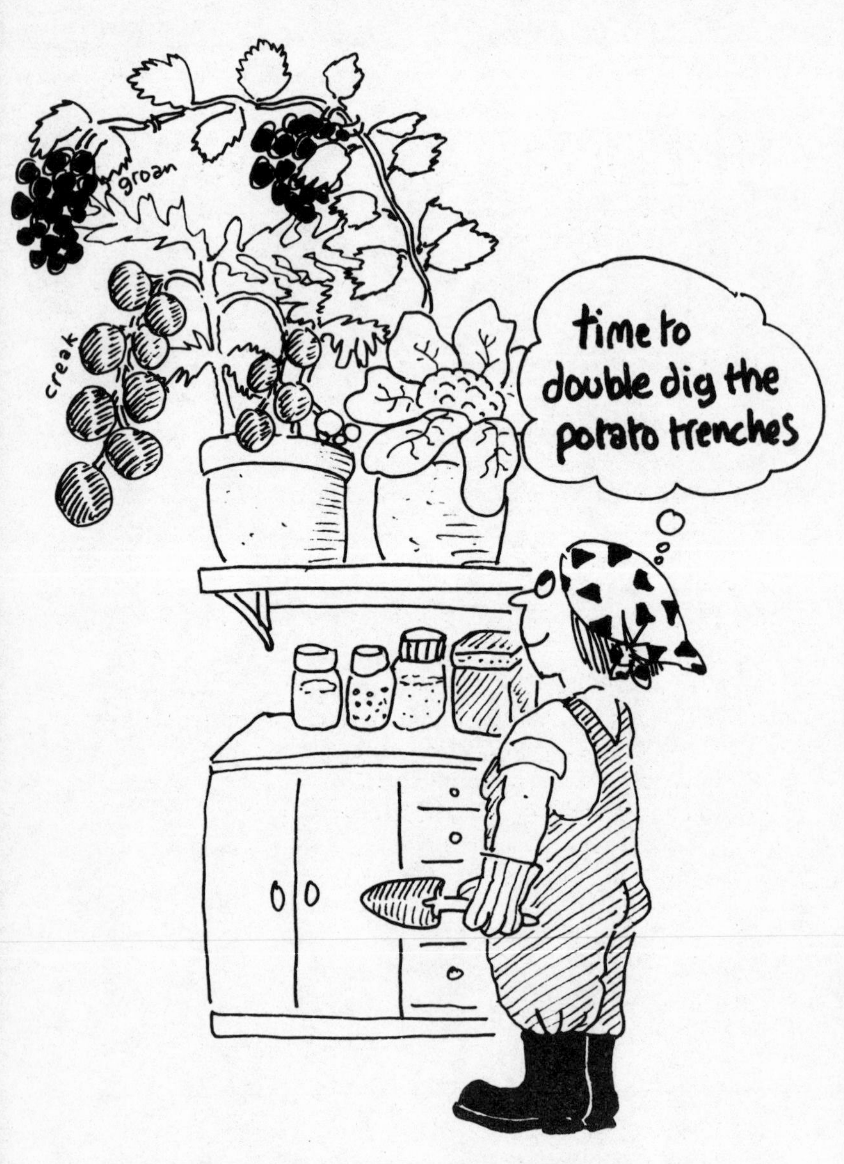

Even if you have only a couple of pots on a shelf . . .

2 Getting a new perspective on food

QUIZ

1 Where do you shop for your food?
2 Do you usually shop during the day or in the evening?
3 What most affects your choice of items?
   a) taste?
   b) nutrition?
   c) price?
4 Do you think advertising has any influence on your choice of product?
5 Do you read labels?
6 If so, do you feel you understand the information given?
7 Have you ever purchased a food item because it was advertised as being low in calories?
8 In an average week, how often do you eat
   a) meat?
   b) fish?
   c) eggs?
   d) pulses?
   e) nuts?
9 Do you grow or make any of your own foods such as
   a) vegetables?
   b) bean sprouts?
   c) bread?
10 If so, do you do so
   a) to save money?
   b) because you consider them nutritionally superior?
   c) to avoid additives?

Catching the customers

An interest in food and awareness of how and why we eat isn't just the prerogative of dieters. During an average lifetime we in the West will consume between twenty and thirty tons of food per person. That's enough to fill a juggernaut. When you think how vital is the role food plays in what you are – not just how you look but in how your body functions, how long you live, even your moods and intelligence – then you might agree that your choice of food should be motivated by more than a catchy commercial or a bargain price.

Up to some forty years ago most of the foods we ate were produced by natural well-established methods in or near the area where we lived, and were eaten whilst still relatively fresh. In other words, they were what we now call wholefoods. And though there is new and growing interest in this simple way of eating, it must be said that the British as a people are still slow to give up old and well-established habits.

Certainly many of us are making small changes: the consumption of fresh vegetables has risen steadily, muesli often replaces fried bacon at the breakfast table, and milkmen are getting more orders for semi-skimmed milk to pour over it. But some seventy percent of the British diet is still made up of processed foods, which means food that has been tinned, frozen, dried, pre-cooked. Irradiation is the latest kind of processing to be marketed, a technique that has been used for some time to sterilise medical instruments. Against the obvious advantages (extending shelf-life, keeping food looking attractive, destroying pathogenic bacteria) come many questions. What will it do to existing pesticide residues, how will it affect nutrients, and how can the law ensure irradiation isn't used to cover up poor quality food?

Most processing methods could, in theory, be used to cover up inferior ingredients, though there are standards set and maintained by the government, and in any case, manufacturers — though principally concerned with making money – do not want to poison their customers. Many of them will point to the advantages of such foods. When once only seasonal and locally available ingredients could be offered, processing has made it possible for us to have an enormous choice of all sorts of foods throughout the year. Their long shelf-life, and the fact that they do not go off, means there is no waste for the manufacturer; hence they help keep his profits healthy. Once purchased, these products can also be kept at home until needed. And – in an age when people are living fuller lives, travelling, taking up hobbies and sports, and spending less time than ever in the kitchen – the convenience aspect of foods that need little more than unwrapping or defrosting and then heating through is obviously an important one.

It's hard not to be tempted.

A walk through one of the vast new supermarkets that are springing up all over the country can be a similar experience to that of being hypnotised. Polished floors, soft music, air conditioning. And row after row of shelves displaying colourful and attractively packaged products, all of which have been designed to catch your eye, to make your hand reach out. In many cases you will find up to half a dozen different makes of the same product.

The plus to the consumer of this competitive way of marketing is that it keeps prices down. There are always special offers to entice you: twenty-five percent extra free, money off your next purchase of the same product, three for the price of two.

End of the corner shop?

Being able to offer such value for money (without sacrificing profits) not only entices customers, but also keeps outside competition to the minimum. Since supermarkets began to appear in cities, towns, even remote villages, the corner shop is becoming a thing of the past. Small retail outlets have to keep their prices higher if they are to stay in business, yet at the same time a slow turnover may mean their products are less fresh, and lack of space means they can offer only a limited choice. In inner-city areas some do still flourish, usually as speciality shops such as delicatessens, or selling ethnic foods, and most of them keep open late into the evening and on

Sundays, which makes them especially appealing to those who cannot shop during the day. Even so, they are a minority group, and the personal contact between shopkeeper and customer that used to make shopping more of a social occasion than a chore is becoming a thing you find only in television commercials.

Whether sold in supermarket or corner shop, all processed foods are now subject to an EEC directive that obliges the manufacturer to indicate any additives either by name or by 'E' number. Though there are also strict rules governing what additives can be used – they must be indispensable, mustn't deceive the customer as to the nature of the food or the quality, and so on – some experts still believe the majority of these are unnecessary. Opinions as to the safety of additives vary enormously from one country to another; in America a more vociferous public has brought about the banning of many that are still widely used in Britain. Artificial colours, usually derived from coal tar, are especially controversial. The fact that these are regularly used to make foods and drinks appeal to children, and the increasing incidence of hyperactivity (and crime, some say) in the young, is a link that is causing concern. Do you read labels? A growing number of shoppers do, though it is doubtful that the average woman or man in the street can make much use of the information given. For example, there is a general belief that all additives are derived from chemicals, yet many colourants are natural in origin. Does that mean they are safe? And antioxidants – these prevent food from going rancid, which is surely a good thing, but the widely used BHA (E320) and BHT (E321) may cause hives as well as hyperactivity. Besides, when a product goes off it is nature's way of saying it shouldn't be eaten, it has passed its best, so antioxidants are actually encouraging us to eat stale food. And though each new additive must be tested for safety before it can be introduced (ones that have been in use for some time are assumed to be safe) there is the question of what happens when they are used in different combinations. Or eaten together with other processed foods that might well contain different additives.

Diet and diesease

Balancing the growth in public concern about such things as additives, the past decade has seen more interest in a positive approach to eating for health. The connection between diet and disease has come under professional scrutiny throughout the world with some sixty–five separate reviews coming to much the same conclusions. Food manufacturers – understandably – have taken the opportunity to turn this increasing awareness to their advantage by adapting their product, or highlighting aspects of it that have previously been overlooked. Thus we now have junk foods such as boiled sweets and soft drinks with added vitamins, refined and fat-laden biscuits turned into 'wholefoods' by the addition of a sprinkling of bran. It must be said that some of the more responsible manufacturers have genuinely improved their products. Ready–to–eat baby foods are now no longer automatically sweetened, crisps are available in low fat varieties, or with the potato skin left on so that they are higher in fibre. But still there is too much misleading flagging on packages which – when backed by advertising – may well increase sales, but does so dishonestly.

Possibly the most over-worked word of the day has been 'natural'. The number of products claiming to be either completely natural, or to offer such benefits as 'natural goodness' or 'a taste of nature' increases daily. It seems likely that the government may soon put restrictions on the use of this word in labelling and advertising, though there will no doubt be many arguments over where these should begin and end.

Running a close second, though, as words that sell, must come 'low calorie'. Manufacturers have long been aware of the British obsession for dieting – and not just the manufacturers of special foods. It doesn't take a genius to see that many conventional foods will sell in considerably larger quantities if dieters are persuaded that they can eat them too – and that this can be done without needing to change the product itself in any way. What is changed is the sales pitch. Promising a low calorie count does the trick without even needing to say lower than what. In many cases a home-prepared version of the same dish would contain even fewer calories. It's quite possible the same product made by a different company may be lower in calories too, but the manufacturers may not have jumped on this particular band waggon. Low is a relative word, and on its own it is meaningless.

Have no doubt about it: the food industry is in the business to make money. Which means it aims to encourage us to eat more. One way in which it hopes to achieve this is by launching nearly a thousand new products every year, backing them with expensive advertising in an effort to convince us that not only will we enjoy eating their product, but that our families and friends will love us more, the sun will always shine, and life will be one long party! Nearly a sixth of all advertising in the UK is spent on promoting food, and employs some of the country's most creative art directors and copywriters to do the job. Though few of these products will still be around two years later, new ones will be ready to take their place.

Beware – minefield!

For the general public, the shopper, people like you and me, finding a way through all these products and promises is about as risky as getting through a minefield. Who do we believe? Are prices fair, and are we getting what we pay for? Should we let price dictate our choice of product anyway, or should we go first for taste? Or nutritional value? How can we judge what nutrients a product contains – or if indeed it has any at all?

And is food safe? Quite apart from doubts about additives there are other dangers associated with the eating of a number of foodstuffs these days, dangers highlighted by the press and too often over-sensationalised, but dangers that are there just the same. Salmonella has been found in a variety of foods, but is particularly prevalent in chicken, some sixty percent of chickens on sale being contaminated. Cases of listeriosis, which have an estimated one in four mortality rate, have been growing in number. Britain is the only country that has bovine spongiform encephalopathy (BSE) – also called mad cow disease – a disease that progressively destroys the brains of cattle, and that has transferred from sheep, where it is known as scrapie. It is almost certain that the habit of adding ground–up sheep carcasses to cattle feed is responsible for allowing the disease to spread this way. Evidence of it has also been found in factory-farmed mink, in zoos, and also in cats, which is not surprising when you consider what pet foods contain. However, it has not been seen in other food-producing animals, though as the disease can take many years to show, and few factory-farmed animals live more than two years, this does not prove they are disease free. No-one knows if the virus can be passed on to humans, though it is certain that we can suffer from infections of a similar type. What *is* known is that normal home cooking cannot be relied upon to destroy the BSE agent.

A very recent effect of all this is just beginning to be observed and commented on, one that appears to be unique to this time in history, and to the affluent West. It is that eating – an activity vital for our survival – is becoming one that is also full of fear.

Fear of food

Food related scares over past centuries may have been common, but they were relatively simple. Would there be enough to eat – or anything at all? That is no longer something that bothers most readers of this book. Instead, food to us has become complicated, the facts changing day by day, one expert giving an opinion and being immediately contradicated by another. And most of the news is bad news. Even when we think we've got it right there will be some little paragraph in a magazine or a newspaper. Fruit, you say. Can't be much wrong with that, can there? Then you read about pesticides used on the fruit tree or bush, techniques used to make the fruit grow bigger, polishes added to make it look good. Or milk, everyone knows milk is a near perfect food. It was – goes the latest thinking – before dairy cows became so sickly that they need to be continually stuffed full of antibiotics and hormones and who knows what else. And what about mad cow disease? Besides, cows are no longer real animals. They're genetic mutants.

Eggs? you say, already knowing the answer. Fish? Nuts?

Add to all this the very real fear (felt by literally millions of people each day) that food makes you fat, and you have the start of a very rare thing – a neurosis that could become an epidemic.

It is hardly surprising that some of the more level minded experts are suggesting that stress caused from worrying about food might well do more harm than the food itself!

Let's go back a few steps.

Why do we eat? The main reason – though one that is usually overlooked – is that food supplies our bodies with the nutrients it needs to keep going. It gives us energy, keeps us warm. After air and water, it is the third most important necessity for the sustaining of life.

Most of us also eat for pleasure. Putting something into the mouth has a calming effect, which is why we give dummies to babies – and why many grown-ups enjoy sucking on a cigarette, pipe or cigar. With food, however, there is the added benefit of taste and texture, particularly if it is something we especially like. We swallow and our hunger pangs subside, and that too feels good.

Another reason for eating is that it is a way of socialising. The family gathering around the kitchen table, the buffet party where you get together with friends, the romantic tête-à-tête over a candlelit table in the corner of your local wine bar – in each case food is an intrinsic part of the occasion, adding to the pleasure of being in the company of people you like or love.

Which brings up another point: feeding people is a very tangible way of showing them you care. The reverse is also true – when someone serves you food they've prepared, you feel flattered, pleased. Nowadays paying for a meal in a restaurant is an alternative way to make the point, and though the personal touch may be missing, the message will get through just as clearly. Pick the right restaurant and you might well enjoy the food too.

By letting fear of food – whether it be for one or more of the many reasons listed above – take away this very basic pleasure, you are denying yourself one of the greatest joys of life. *You are denying yourself.*

The three-way path

So what can you do? There is no one simple answer, but by changing your whole approach to the subject of food and dieting, you may well find a way through the minefield . . . and actually begin enjoying food again.

The three-way path is simple, logical, and easier to follow than you may think.

1. Learn which foods will do you most good (and least harm), stock up with them, throw out everything else.
2. Vary them as much as possible.
3. Relax and enjoy!

If this sounds like another list of rules, of do's and don'ts, it isn't intended to be. Think of it more as a framework on which you can build an eating pattern that suits your lifestyle, your personal tastes and preferences – and your personality too. But it must be admitted that you may well need to make some changes before you start.

Changing attitudes

Changes can be approached in a number of ways. Many nationalities actually enjoy the challenge of change – Americans, for example, are generally open to the adventure of trying something new (definite links with their ancestors here!) The British are traditionalists and proud of it, used to holding fast to the established way of doing things. This means that change tends to be seen as something to be avoided; it will require effort, it may be painful. It could even be an absolute disaster. Certainly change for the sake of it is foolish, and there is much to be conserved and valued from times gone past. Just the same, change is life. Something that never changes is static, inert, fixed. In other words, it is dead.

Your attitude to change will very much affect your ability to cope with it. As with most things in life, if you anticipate problems you'll be sure to find them. Alternatively, you can take a positive approach. Tell yourself that this is going to be a learning experience, one that will not only improve your health and be enjoyable, but that will mean an end to dieting once and for all!

If dieting has become such a habit that you suspect you will feel strange – even unhappy – if you're *not* on a diet, ask yourself why you feel this way. Does dieting give you a purpose in life? Are all your friends dieting, and do you feel you'll no longer belong if you break the habit? Do you feel frightened at the idea of letting go, not having to hold back all the time, as though you might eat so much you'll blow up like a balloon? It might help to talk your thoughts through with someone who will listen and understand, either someone close to you or a trained counsellor.

Remember too that although it is true that our eating habits are instilled in all of us way back in our childhood, they do adapt as we grow older. If this wasn't so, many of us would still be craving jam tarts and jelly (some of us do, of course). But most of us have learned to like at least some new foods, have experimented with foreign dishes, or dishes made with ingredients that are unfamiliar. Often our introduction to such foods came when holidaying in another country, or dining at a restaurant. We think of these as pleasurable experiences. Discovering wholefoods can be just as pleasurable.

Calories out for the count

The first thing to do – which for many will be a relief – is to forget about calories. A calorie is the unit by which energy is measured. It refers to the amount of heat needed to raise the temperature of a gram of water by one degree centigrade. Nowadays food is measured in kilocalories, yet the older term is still the one most widely used. Diets relying on calorie reduction are the most common, and even those that claim to be different tend to be based on cutting your intake of calories, even though this fact may be hidden under a multitude of disguises. And it's true that if you reduce your consumption of calories to a low enough level, you *will* lose weight – for a while, at least.

Most dieters are good at counting calories. If they're chronic dieters they may have an inbuilt computer: feed in the food name, up will flash the calorie count. There are two reasons why counting calories this way is unwise. Firstly, the relevance of adjusting your calorie intake is closely linked with your metabolic rate, which is the speed at which your body uses the energy it needs for all your body processes – renewing cells, digesting food and the working of other vital organs, and physical activity. Note the word – *your* metabolic rate.

This not only varies from person to person, but though you will tend to start out in life with – for example – a slow or fast rate, this will not necessarily remain static. Changes in your lifestyle can affect it. Or you can choose to change it yourself by eating more, which will speed it up, or less, when it will slow down for a time. Your metabolism is like a safety valve. Its function is to keep your body in balance despite fluctuations in the fuel you give it and the things you require it to do.

It follows, then, that any chart promising you a certain weight loss if you keep to a certain number of calories per day, cannot be accurate. Or to put it another way: it may be right for some dieters, but certainly not for everyone. There is even a theory going about that the majority of 'overweight' people have gained the extra pounds not because of taking in too many calories – some surveys show, in fact, that they often eat less than thin people. The causes of overweight are much more complex, says this theory. The Royal College of Physicians, talking about obesity studies carried out over the past fifty years, said there seems little doubt that there is a general trend for both men and women to become heavier and presumably fatter. Why should you try to 'diet' when the very experts you're trying to follow are moving the goal posts?

But an even better reason for giving up counting calories is that it is tiresome, a bore. For you and also for everyone around you! Choosing foods you know to be lowish in calories, and that you enjoy eating, is one thing. Forcing yourself to eat things you don't like because they have few calories is another thing altogether. How many dieters come to have nightmares about cottage cheese? Don't forget that *all* food contains calories. The reason many vegetables are listed as 'permissible' is that they contain a lot of water, but in theory, if you could eat enough of them you could go over your calorie allowance even on celery sticks. Just as ridiculous as eating what you don't like is the business of weighing and measuring everything. How can a meal be a pleasure when instead of using a fork you approach it with scales and a ruler?

If you can't choose what foods to eat by their calories, of course, you have to find some other way. How about taste? What about freshness and naturalness? How about eating things that make you feel full of energy?

Back to nature

Although nutritionalists may have differing opinions on so many of the details as to what we should and shouldn't be eating, it is amazing on how many points they do agree. The basic advice is consistent and simple.

1. Eat less saturated fats.
2. Eat more fresh vegetables and fruit for their vitamins, minerals and fibre content.
3. Get your protein from pulses, seeds, nuts and wholegrains.
4. As far as possible, avoid all processed foods.

In other words, go back to nature!

The easiest way to cut right back on saturated fats is to give up eating meat. Do this and you'll also reduce your intake of a whole range of 'additives': drugs given to allay the diseases that are endemic when animals are intensively reared in unnatural and unhygienic conditions, tranquillisers given to calm them, growth boosting hormones used to increase farmers' profits, plus things such as polyphosphate salts (widely used to increase the water content of meat and fish).

In Britain, the consumption of red meat has dropped drastically in recent years and fish has once again become popular, though quite apart from the ethics of whether or not it is right to kill, there is also concern about just how healthy fish is these days. Without doubt it is low in fat, but with our seas becoming increasingly polluted, the concern is more than mere fancy. A report in 1990 suggested that with so much untreated sewage and rubbish being dumped often only a short distance from the coast, seafood should be eaten with caution. Illnesses that could be contracted from it, the report warned, include hepatitis and cholera.

If vegetarians used to be considered cranks, they're not any longer. Nowadays there are well over three million of them in Britain alone (plus another hundred thousand vegans), all proof that giving up flesh foods isn't such a difficult thing to do. As their numbers grow, so does the selection of alternatives offered by food manufacturers to fill the protein gap.

Dairy produce is an obvious source of protein and many other nutrients. Use free-range eggs (those from factory farmed chickens cannot be called a natural food), some milk if you must (preferably goat's milk from animals still farmed on a small scale), cheese, yogurt. Try also tofu, a soya curd that has twice the protein of meat, four times that of eggs, lots of vitamins and minerals and no cholesterol. There are also various textured soya products that have the consistency of meat; use them in sauces, lasagnes and curries if you really miss the real thing. Protein is made up from twenty-three amino acids, eight of which are considered essential (nine for children). It used to be claimed that flesh foods were the very best source of protein. Wholegrains such as brown rice, oats, barley, millet, rye, and wheat (mostly consumed in the form of flour) all contain some amino acids, but no single one contains the eight essentials. The answer is to combine foods so that together they will give you all the amino acids you need, and in the right balance. This is not as complicated as it sounds. All you have to do is remember to serve your grain with a food from another category – which is something you'd probably do anyway. For example, add pulses (chili beans on rice would be perfect), nuts (peanut butter with toast), seeds (tahini with pita bread). Or – if you feel a need for some dairy produce – add grated cheese, a dollop of yogurt, an egg to bind your ingredients. And if it sounds as though you'll still end up consuming less protein than if you'd eaten a slice of steak – you're right. Just as well, as it is now suspected we don't need nearly as much protein as was thought a few decades ago. Any excess protein is used for energy rather than for producing new cells and repairing, which makes it not only wasteful (carbohydrates do the job better, and are cheaper), but any that isn't used must be either stored or removed, both alternatives putting an unnecessary strain on the body.

Package deal value

There's another big plus when you take most of your food from plants. You could think of it as a package deal, and one that's especially good value. Nutritionalists tell us to eat more fibre; plant foods are full of natural fibre, and in the right form and balance for us to utilise it with the minimum effort. Nutritionalists say vitamins and minerals are important; plant foods are their best source. Nutritionalists say increase your consumption of polyunsaturated oils (the kind that not only don't clog your arteries, but actually help to clear them); these almost all come from plants.

Though it might sound as if this way of eating is going to need just as much attention to detail as going on a diet, it won't, not once you've got into the swing of things. Nor will it be dull, boring, difficult to follow – and it won't leave you feeling hungry either.

Remember the three-way path. First step is to throw out all those foods you know to be unhealthy, and to replace them with wholefoods. The lists below will cover the basics you might need – you can add to them as you get more used to this new way of cooking.

For your cupboard
Dried pulses such as chick peas, butter beans, aduki beans, kidney beans, lentils, soya beans, split peas
Grains such as brown rice, barley, rye, millet, oats, bulgar wheat
Wholemeal flour
Dried fruits
Nuts such as hazels, almonds, walnuts, brazils, peanuts
Seeds such as sesame, sunflower, pumpkin, poppy
Yeast extract or miso
Sea salt
Tamari soya sauce
Ground black pepper
Spices
Dried herbs
Vegetable oil – preferably cold-pressed
Olive oil if liked
Nut butters
Tahini
Tomato purée
Sea vegetables such as kelp, wakame, nori
Gelling ingredient such as agar-agar
Wholegrain biscuits such as those made with rye or oats
Dried wholegrain pastas
Cider vinegar
Soya milk
Raw cane sugar
Honey

For your fridge
Tofu
Tempeh
Polyunsaturated or vegan margarine
Live yogurt – dairy or soya
Vegetarian cheddar cheese
Cow's or goat's milk
Vegetables as available
Sprouted beans or seeds

Tofu or egg mayonnaise

You do not, of course, need all these ingredients to start with, but the better your selection, the more creative your cooking will be. And once you've got used to the basic idea of using wholefoods, do be creative. To start with, try some of the recipes given at the end of this book. There are many other books available on wholefood cookery; look too at books of recipes from other countries and cultures. A large proportion of the world's population base their cookery on grains and vegetables, use little or no meat, and yet their cuisines are anything but dull!

Whilst learning to cook different dishes or experimenting with your own ideas, do try to vary the ingredients you reach for. Because cooking is a habit, we all tend to have favourite recipes, ingredients which we pick up automatically when we go shopping. Even though you will be using ingredients that are close to nature, in this day and age many of them will still have come into contact with some pesticides, or will have been grown from soil that was treated with chemicals – this is inevitable. By varying the ingredients you cook with you will be adding interest to your meals, whilst at the same time minimising the possibility of any harmful effects.

Another way to do this is to shop in different places. If you have a local wholefood shop, you are lucky. There you will no doubt find an excellent selection of top quality foods grown with care and attention, many of them organic. But nowadays it is also possible to buy wholefoods in local shops; a delicatessen, for example, might well stock such continental favourites as tahini, hummus, wholemeal pita bread. And supermarkets too – very sensitive to public demand – are now selling organic vegetables, wholegrain products, pulses, tofu, goat's milk, and many other such foods. If you can't find what you want, ask for the manager and request that it is stocked. If he knows what he's doing – and he wouldn't be a manager if he didn't – he will get it in for you.

One point about shopping that is rarely considered. If at all possible, shop when you are not in too much of a rush, and when you are not tired. Though you will not need to read many labels (you'll eliminate that fuss by concentrating on foods that contain no or very few 'E' additives anyway), you will still need to have time to shop with care. Hurry and you may well pick up the wrong item by mistake, or substitute one of inferior quality. Shop when tired and you may find yourself suddenly craving a chocolate bar or gooey cake. One will do you little harm, but white sugar is addictive, so one may well lead to another. If you've worked hard to get into the habit of eating healthily, it's a shame to break it just because you couldn't shop at a time when you were in a more positive frame of mind.

Do it yourself

If you can produce some of your own foods, so much the better. The smallest garden will yield a considerable crop of vegetables if you plan carefully, and not only will you be able to pick them minutes before you use them (which gives a whole new meaning to the word *fresh*) but you'll know for sure that they are free from any kind of chemicals. Even if you have only a window box or a couple of pots on a shelf, you can grow a variety of food plants. Herbs are especially suitable. Sadly, these are still not used as widely in Britain as they are in many parts of the world, where they play an essential role in both flavouring food and aiding digestion. Any surplus herbs can be dried and kept for use later. Remember that you need far less of dried herbs as their flavour is more concentrated.

Another food you can easily produce at home is sprouted beans, seeds and grains. The results will vary enormously depending on which variety you choose, and can be added to salads, used in soups and casseroles, or stir-fried.

In fact, anyone with the interest – and time to spare – can produce a cornucopia of good wholesome foods at home. You can bake your own bread, biscuits, cakes, make jams, nut butters, soft cheese, yogurt. The important thing is to feel not that you *ought* to but that you *want* to. If not, buy the things you need.This new way of eating is based on discovering for yourself the pleasure it can give, easing yourself into it rather than setting rules and threatening yourself with punishments. That's how most slimming diets may work, but you've finished with them. From now on you're aiming to learn how to enjoy food – without pressure, without guilt. Using pleasure-power instead of will-power, you could say. In many ways this final step on the three-way path is the most important.

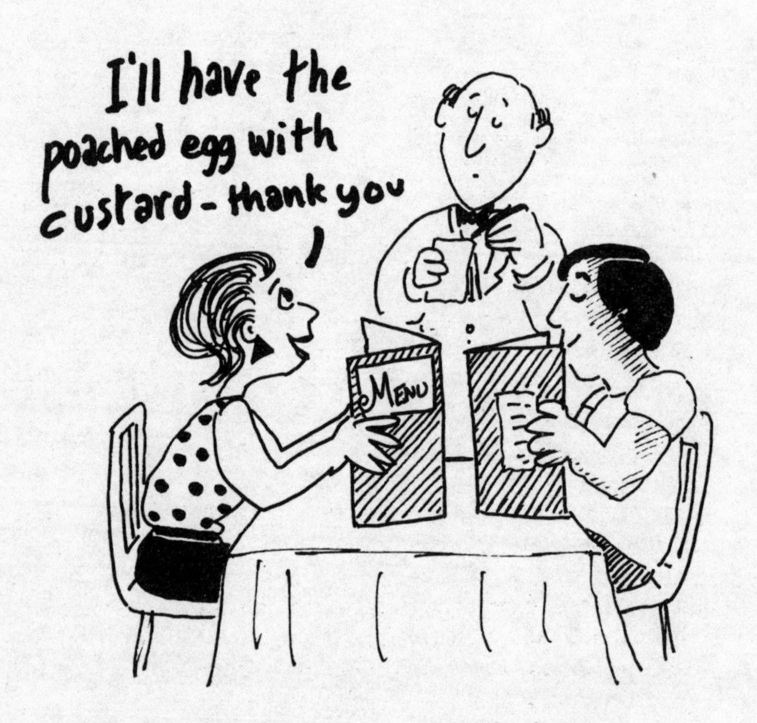

Foods with snob appeal are constantly changing . . .

3 *A* matter of taste

QUIZ

1 Do you crave chocolate or sugary foods
- a) when tired?
- b) when feeling low?
- c) when it's cold?

2 Do you associate sweet things with special treats, holiday occasions, romance, going to the cinema and so on?

3 Once started on something sweet, do you find yourself unable to stop?

4 Or – when having a snack – is your preference for salty foods such as crisps and olives?

5 What about texture? Do you tend to choose soft, smooth foods like ice cream, mashed potatoes, pâté?

6 Or do crunchy foods such as toast, celery or nuts give you more satisfaction?

7 Have you ever anticipated eating something – really looked forward to it – and then found it didn't come up to expectation?

8 Do you enjoy experimenting with new foods, or prefer to stick with those you know?

9 Have you sometimes suspected that certain foods might be
- a) making you or your children hyperactive?
- b) giving you headaches?
- c) affecting you physically in another way?

10 When eating a meal do you prefer to leave the table feeling
- a) slightly hungry?
- b) just about full?
- c) as though you couldn't eat another thing?

The sniff test

In a restaurant, or at a buffet party, most people go for the same foods time and again. Have you ever asked yourself why this is? You like the taste, you'll probably say. And certainly taste is an important factor.

The sense of taste is localised in the tongue which is covered in numerous minute elevations called papillae that give it its rough feel. The end-organs for the sense of taste are gathered in clumps, mostly at the side and base of the tongue. These are your taste buds. Surprisingly, they can only detect four primary tastes: bitter, sweet, salt and sour.

It is through your sense of smell that you 'taste' most foods. This very delicate sense can pick up a wider variety of odours than anyone could possibly classify; in fact, it's estimated that it is about 10,000 times more acute than your sense of taste. So when you have a head cold and the nasal mucous membrane is inflamed, it may seem as though you can't taste your food, when the truth is that you can't *smell* it. This may also explain why people with permanently impaired olfactory senses quite often also have poor appetites.

But taste is only part of the story.

As already pointed out, eating is one of the most habit-bound of activities. How to obtain nourishment is probably one of the very first lessons we learn, and though this starts out as an instinctive need to do something about the hunger pangs, it soon changes. Our parents – most often our mother in particular – have a lot to do with the way we eat for the rest of our lives. It is the foods we are given during those early years that set the pattern, and not just what we ate but when and in what circumstances. Unvaried meals served at regular times might well result in a reluctance, in later years, to be at all flexible about food. If we were not allowed to leave the table until our plates were scraped clean, we might well – even as adults – continue to feel obliged to eat everything put in front of us (which may mean we get into the habit of eating more than our bodies need or even want).

Who we usually dined with and the atmosphere at the table can also colour our feelings about food in later years. If childhood meals tended to be happy occasions, this will stay with us. Meals always eaten in a rush can lead to feelings of guilt or indulgence about taking time to enjoy eating. If, however, the coming together of the family around a table invariably meant friction and arguments, we may well never really enjoy mealtimes again.

The mother who used food to comfort a child, or maybe as a substitute for attention, will have instilled a need for food that will automatically arise in times of distress or loneliness. If food was withheld as a bribe or punishment, that could result in overeating as a belated compensation, though this type of behaviour in adults could also be a way of asserting him or herself, of breaking free. Psychiatrists and counsellors are dealing with a growing number of eating disorders based on childhood experiences, though probably the majority of adults come through relatively unscathed.

The need to belong

There is more learning to be done along the way however. As soon as a child is old enough to read and watch television, other (and very powerful) influences come onto the scene. Manufacturers are well aware of the importance of catching their customers early. It is during their teens that many youngsters go through the phase of wanting to look like their friends, do what their friends are doing, fit in with the crowd. Advertisements designed to latch on to this need are especially effective; think of commercials for Coca Cola and McDonalds. Fast foods, take-aways, snacks munched whilst on the move – many young people, especially those who live in cities, know no other way of eating today. In the trade they are known as 'grazers'. Again, they may well be setting habits that will last well into the future.

Advertising has much to do also with our tendency to associate sweet things with celebrations, special occasions, the giving of gifts. It cannot claim responsibility for initiating the idea though. For centuries sugar was a luxury item, not just in Britain but throughout the world, and was therefore only used on high days and holidays. Even now sweetmeats are offered to revered deities as part of religious ceremonies in many Eastern countries. Closer to home, a box of chocolates is presented as a sign of love to girlfriends, wives, mothers, children – though less commonly to men. Just the same, it seems to be considered quite acceptable for men to help eat them, and a craving for sugary things is equally common in both sexes. Interesting to note that consuming sweet foods seems to have become the Eighth Deadly Sin – which makes it just as desirable an activity as the other seven!

Food snobbery

If sweets are considered deliciously naughty, thus giving the impression that whoever eats them is wild and free-thinking, there are other foods that give a completely different but seemingly equally desirable impression. These are foods you rarely find in people's homes, unless they are being served at a dinner party, one intended to impress. Mostly they are consumed in restaurants where the prices – if shown – reflect the fact that these are something very special. Such gourmet foods might include pheasant, venison, oysters, snails in garlic butter. Most of them are meat or fish dishes which – like sugar – were once the prerogative of the wealthy upper classes. As one way to appear to be affluent, discriminating, sophisticated (even if you're not) is to mimic those who are, the eating of such foods presumably enhances the image of the diner. Which explains the importance of doing it in public. And if many of them are very much an acquired taste – few of us grow up on these more exotic foods, unless our families were wealthy, or our fathers gamekeepers – it seems that's a small price to pay.

The increase in such gourmets, and their obvious willingness to spend whatever is necessary to maintain their image, has led to a whole industry that supplies not just the foods but the wines to go with them, the highly specialised tableware, plus numerous guides as to which little restaurant in which little back street is the 'in' place this year. Such people are, in many ways, displaying much the same need to belong, to prove themselves, as the teenager hanging around outside McDonalds with a burger and coke.

Foods with snob appeal are constantly changing, some losing appeal, others taking their place. Because of the growing market for venison, deer have become one of the most recent animals to be specifically farmed for their meat. Inevitably, farming on a large scale does tend to bring prices down; chicken, not so long ago, was something you had on Sundays, if you were lucky, whereas now most British people can afford to eat it every day. It is therefore no longer a luxury food, and those who set trends must find something new. Amongst the more recent additions to the in-people's menus are wild boar, kangaroo steaks, dormice.

But if the way we eat is set to a large extent by the way we are brought up, and then moulded by the society in which we live, there is one other element that is rarely considered, though it's an important one. That is each person's very different physical and mental make-up. A closer look at the foods you prefer can in fact reveal some truths that might surprise you. Of course your choice at any given moment would be dictated to some extent at least by external circumstances. Weather for example has a strong influence on the foods we fancy at different times of year. Hot soup on a winter's day is a most appealing idea; on a sizzling summer day it's probably the last thing you'd choose. Then again, conditions in the place where you are to eat may change all that. Cold outside it may be, but if the central heating is going full blast you may still not fancy soup.

Your body's nutritional needs will also affect your choice, and they will depend very much on what you were doing immediately before you started to eat, what state of health you're in, and such things.

Links between food and personality

Still, we all have a tendency to go for certain foods, and psychiatrists can see definite links between this and our personality types.

What would you say is *your* favourite food, or type of food? Think about it. Imagine you've been out walking all day and have not eaten a thing since breakfast. Or that you've been in bed with flu, and your appetite has just returned and you're starving. Or that you've had a terrible day at the office.

Soft-textured, smooth foods are comforters. They slide down with no effort, make you feel good, special. Many of these foods are associated with childhood, or with being nursed back from ill health. Anyone who eats them all the time is indicating a very basic need for love, a longing to be cosseted and pampered, say the experts.

Chocolates, sweets and very sweet foods will probably appeal to the same people, though they are not just comforting but can also be seen as a reward for something achieved, or compensation when things go wrong.

It is suggested that a tendency to go for crunchy foods shows an inner anger or tension. Biting hard into a stick of celery, a crispbread or a handful of nuts can give relief in much the say way as hammering away at a punchball.

Heavy, stodgy foods give a feeling of satiety. They also draw blood to the stomach in order to help the digestive process, which in turn tends to make you sleepy. A desire for plates of pasta, suet puddings and rice pilafs can be a way of switching off, opting out. Salty and highly spiced foods, though, can indicate quite the opposite – a need for stimulation, variety, a challenge maybe. As in life, too much spicy food does in fact desensitise the taste buds so that the full flavour cannot be appreciated, resulting in a need for foods even more highly flavoured. Salt has much the same effect.

It is hard of course to extricate mental from physical needs when it comes to food. All of us are not only highly complex, but we're also individuals with very different bodies and lifestyles. And in the end the only person who can tell you what foods will work best for you – is you yourself.

Allergies on the increase

Even so, it's not always easy to judge accurately if an ingredient suits you, even if it is considered to be nutritious and natural. Allergies are a major problem of recent years, sufferers reporting a wide variety of symptoms including migraines and headaches, breathing problems, itching and skin rashes, nausea and vomiting, irritability, anxiety, and many more. Though probably the majority are associated with the increasing use of additives in food, some allergies can be traced back to basic and seemingly innocent ingredients such as wheat, milk, cheese, bananas, citrus fruits. New production methods, however, often involve the use of chemicals even for these foods, which may explain the increase in allergic reaction to them.

Ironically, many allergies can actually cause a craving for the very same food that is creating the problem. Recent research in America has suggested a link between iron deficiences and food cravings, but this theory has still to be examined more thoroughly. Meanwhile, the only course to take if you suspect you may be allergic to one or more foods is to try to identify exactly which food or foods are causing the allergy. Though the medical profession is gradually (if grudgingly) accepting such problems might be real rather than imagined, many doctors are still disinclined to do much more than prescribe antihistamines, nosedrops and nasal sprays, steroids, salves and creams. With restricted time and finances, there is probably little more they *can* do. Not surprisingly, self-help groups have proliferated in recent years, and these will give practical advice as well as encouragement to help you track down culprits that you need to avoid.

Sweets and chocolates can be a major cause of such problems. Certainly they are enjoyable. Take chocolate, for example. Emotionally it can cheer you up, comfort you, be a morale booster. It also contains beta phenylethylamine which is a mood lifting chemical occurring naturally in the brain, and that accounts for the feeling of being on a high. So chocolate gives you a buzz. And with all those calories to warm you on the coldest day, it's small wonder chocolate is so popular! But it also contains not only stimulants that can be addictive, but refined carbohydrates that give an instant energy boost that the body reacts to by pumping out insulin. This brings your blood sugar level down so effectively that it may well drop even lower than it was to start with – and so you crave more chocolate.

This doesn't necessarily mean you have to give up chocolate, either for health reasons, or because of weight. What it does mean is that you should understand it for what it is and does. Add to that an awareness of why you feel you want or need to eat it, and you will be making an informed choice. Being informed is important in all aspects of our daily life, yet so often we muddle through being swept along by forces outside our control, shrugging our shoulders when things go wrong, blaming it on bad luck. Because the way you eat is so very important to your health and happiness, isn't it worth making the effort to learn as much you can about just why you eat the way you do?

Is food your purpose in life?

Physically we all need food. Emotionally, though, our needs may vary enormously. To some people, food is a purpose in life. Eating is one of the most pleasurable things they do, and each minute of the day is spent either thinking about food, shopping for or preparing food, or eating it. Such a person may be a gourmet, a food snob who seeks out and raves about certain delicacies whilst considering most foods fit only for pigs. Or he or she may be a gourmand. The gourmand never turns down the offer of seconds, can't resist scraping those last few spoonsful from the serving dish, and would feel cheated if he or she had to leave the table feeling anything less than satiated, if not bloated.

An over-simplification might be to describe the gourmet as someone who likes to be seen eating, and a gourmand as someone who likes simply to eat. But though the traditional picture of happy-go-lucky chubbies tucking into cream cakes might still hold true in some cases – and if they *are* happy, that's all well and good – many people who eat continually are secret eaters, merely picking at food in public, waiting until they're alone to get down to the serious business. It is this type of eating that can become an obsession.

It is likely that anyone who has an over-reliance on food is trying to compensate for something that is missing or wrong in their lives. They see food as something on which to focus, always looking forward to the next meal or snack, removing themselves from the present moment and anything in it that might be distressing, annoying, demanding. When that food fails to come up to expectations – as is invariably the case – they simply transfer their attention to the next meal. Food can never really satisfy them because it is not food they need. If you feel this description fits you, it might be worth considering getting professional help. Trying forcibly to change your feelings about food is a waste of time. Many if not most eating disorders are a symptom of a problem that may well have nothing at all to do with food. It is only by tracking right back to the roots of this problem, digging them up and examining them closely, that you can hope to change your eating habits for any longer than a day or two.

A mouthful of straw

What about people who don't like food? Because the majority of those with food-related problems tend to overeat, we are likely to forget about those – and there is a surprisingly large number of them – who suffer from a complete lack of interest in food. Not only do they dislike shopping and cooking, but some of them have very genuine problems with actually eating too. Chewing can make them feel like they have a mouthful of straw – and have you ever tried to swallow straw? Part of this may be due to their general health being below par which – when linked with lack of excercise – can result in a poor appetite. As already said, damaged taste buds can lead to food tasting bland and uninteresting – and these buds can be affected by eating too much salt, or highly spiced foods, and by drinking very hot liquids amongst other things. Smoking also has an effect on your ability to taste. The fact that people who give up smoking often put on weight, at least at first, is assumed to be because they need to have something else in their mouths to take the place of the cigarette. It seems reasonable to assume that another reason may well have something to do with their discovering just how good food can really taste!

As with those who have large appetites, there is nothing wrong with eating little and being thin, providing enough food is eaten to supply the nutrients and energy needed. If this is your problem, all you have to do is ask yourself how you feel. Are you sleeping well? Do you have enough energy to do the things you have to do, and maybe a little to spare? How often do you go down with colds and other minor ailments?

Nutrition is about health, and if you are well there is no need to try to force yourself to eat more. The theory is much the same as with the chronic dieter: declare war on your body and it will fight back!

Most people probably fall somewhere between loving and hating food. Yet even they divide into a number of categories. There are those who stick rigidly to the same foods, probably those they grew up with, refusing to be tempted to try anything different with the excuse that they know what they like. Most likely their whole lives are governed by this same cautious attitude. Though it's easy to assume they're in their later years and therefore somehow entitled to be set in their ways, it's surprising how many young people have the same closed minds to both food and life. They are usually strongly influenced by their parents and might well also live in small and insular communities. If they have a local Indian restaurant, you can be sure its most popular dish will be omelette and chips. Such a strong desire for the familiar is understandable. Familiarity may sometimes breed contempt, but it's safe, undemanding, it doesn't require you to take risks nor even to think too much. Yet in an age when walls are tumbling and borders opening, and for the first time in human history people are thinking of themselves as inhabitants of Planet Earth above all else, it seems sad not to be part of it.

A taste for adventure

What, then, of those who are always wanting to try something different? These are the friends who are first to discover a new restaurant, who buy recipe books of cuisines from around the world, who think chop sticks and pasta making machines are standard kitchen equipment. And forget about reading labels! It's the products with labels in foreign languages they go for, the more exotic-sounding the better. Though an adventurous approach to cooking must be a good thing, a desperate yearning for novelty can become as numbing as a diet of the same thing day after day. Someone who eats only exotica will be missing out on the pleasure that can be derived from eating such simple foods as a slice of fresh bread, a newly picked apple, brown rice cooked to perfection and topped with nothing more than a knob of butter.

The secret, once again, is variety. Don't get into eating habits that end up being as restrictive as strait-jackets.

And one final thought on knowing yourself and understanding your eating habits. When is enough enough? Meals, especially those shared with friends or family, can least for literally hours. We think of them as social occasions. In other parts of the world they can go on for days, especially when the occasion is a wedding, or even a funeral. Pleasant though such meals may be, there is a tendency to keep eating simply because you are seated at a table and there is something on it waiting to be consumed. Worse still, conversation may be non-stop and there's a good chance that after the first few delicious mouthfuls you'll hardly notice what you're eating anyway; certainly you'll be deriving little pleasure from the food itself. If such occasions are rare, they can do little harm. But don't let eating this way become a habit.

To know when you've eaten enough you have to concentrate. At the beginning of a meal you may find food tastes especially good. Midway through it you're still enjoying the tastes and textures, though you're no longer so hungry. There will come a point when you've had enough, when not only your appetite has gone, but your stomach feels comfortably full. Don't let other circumstances tell you when you should stop eating; listen to your body and decide for yourself. A gargantuan meal to one person will be a snack to another. Instead of following examples set by others, or eating everything on your plate because it is there, or because it's going to have to be paid for anyway, stop and think. Say no thank you to more if you don't want it. If you're in company, learn to feel at ease even when you're the only one who has finished eating. Discover the art of pushing your chair away from the table.

Taking time to carefully analyse not just what you eat, but why you eat the way you do and how it makes you feel, may seem like a lot of work. It is. But it will be worth it. What you discover will give you an insight into both your emotional and physical needs. It should help you to know yourself a little better, maybe even to like yourself more. Then put this knowledge to use by learning to use wholesome natural foods to satisfy your needs – and don't be surprised if you feel better than you ever have before.

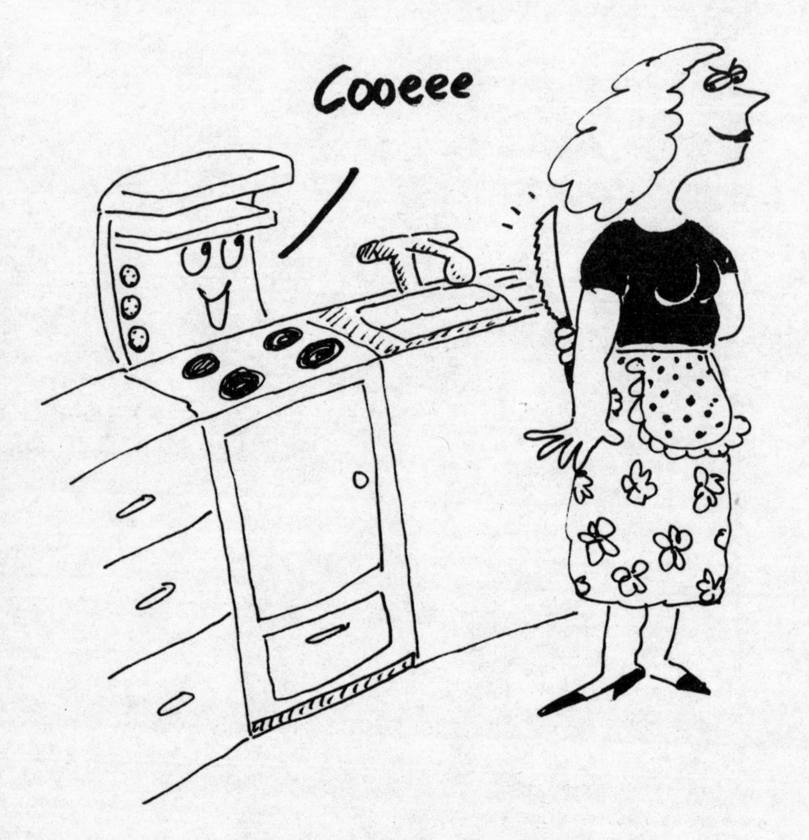

Hate cooking? You're not alone

4 *P*roblems, problems

QUIZ

1 To start your day do you
  a) eat a large cooked breakfast?
  b) have cereal or toast and coffee?
  c) go without anything?

2 If you are at home during the day, do you
  a) eat a snack lunch?
  b) not eat a meal but nibble?
  c) sit down to a proper meal?

3 If you work away from home and take a packed lunch, what does it usually consist of?

4 If business lunches are a regular feature of your working day, do they occur
  a) once a week?
  b) twice a week?
  c) more often?

5 Do such lunches include alcohol?

6 Does the thought of preparing a meal each day
  a) give you pleasure?
  b) count as just another chore?
  c) bore or even depress you?

7 Are you in the habit of inviting people to dinner?

8 Or does your idea of a pleasant evening with friends usually mean going out to the restaurant?

9 Do you buy take-away meals
  a) most days?
  b) now and again?
  c) never?

10 Are you reluctant – or unable – to spend more than the absolute minimum on food?

Taking responsibility

You may have resolved to make the change, to take responsibility for your own health and body by taking a positive approach to food. This may mean changes, but that's alright. You're determined. You've thought too about your emotional as well as physical needs, and have a pretty good idea what they are. You may even have made a start, had a go at a couple of new recipes, thrown out some of the ingredients you're going to ban from your kitchen from now on, replaced them with things you're looking forward to trying.

Making the decision is the first step, and it's a big one. Just the same, few things in life go smoothly. Unless you're exceptionally lucky, sooner or later you're sure to come up against a problem or two. And even small problems can seem like giants if they catch you unawares. Thinking about them in advance – and deciding how you'll overcome them if they *do* crop up – may well make the difference between success, and throwing the whole thing out and going back to the dieting war!

Time for a change?

The working woman is very much a phenomenon of the times. Better education opportunities are partly responsible. Add to that a growing (if grudging!) willingness amongst employers to admit that women can do most jobs just as well as men, and the result is that the majority of women do, at some time in their lives, go out to work. Youngsters often spend their first few years after leaving school in employment, many of them carrying on after getting married. More recently there has been a trend for women to return to work once their children have started school, or when they have grown up and left home.

Yet at the same time the bulk of the responsibility for running the home still rests on the shoulders of women. Much as equality of the sexes may be a popular subject for magazines, research has recently shown that men – though they may help out in the home more than they used to – still see the house as a woman's territory. Whilst it's expected that the husband, at the end of a hard day at the office, will collapse in front of the television, feet up on the sofa, his working wife is more likely to be making the beds and finishing the ironing.

Of course it's hard to keep going under such circumstances, let alone make major changes. Your new way of eating will eventually give you more stamina, more energy, but meanwhile you're going to have to be determined. Start with breakfast. Maybe you have no time to eat? No appetite? For many years dieticians have been extolling the benefits of a large breakfast. After a night of fasting, they say, and before a day of activity, we should refuel. Though the logic is clear to see – and though the British breakfast, complete with fried eggs, bread and bacon, is still obligatory at seaside boarding houses – the idea of a big meal first thing in the morning doesn't appeal to everyone. Some people find it positively stomach churning! And it seems obvious that even though we may not have eaten for some twelve hours, few of us wake up ravenously hungry. Time (or rather the lack of it) is another consideration. If you're off out to work, or about to take the children to school, or walk the dog, or have an exercise class at ten, it's unlikely you'll be able to eat a large breakfast. Nor will you have time to cook it, and even less to wash up afterwards.

On the other hand, the traditional breakfast of busy people and dieters – a cup of black coffee – is bad news. Certainly the caffeine will give you the jolt you may need to get you into action, but it won't provide the nourishment to keep you going past that first hour or so, neither will it calm your nerves, nor help you say no to a doughnut for elevenses! Much better to go for one of the many concoctions that can be whisked together in a minute, drinks made with milk, yogurt or tofu mixed with fruit juices, sweetened if necessary with honey or raw cane sugar. Creamed coconut, pineapple juice and a pinch of spice is a real taste of the tropics! For extra goodness you can add wheat germ, brewers yeast, ground nuts. Essences such as vanilla or peppermint could be used to vary the flavour, or try carob powder for a drink with all the flavour of chocolate but none of the addictive qualities.

Though quick to make and consume, mixtures of this kind can be as nutritious as you choose to make them, and at least you won't leave the house feeling ravenous! A wire whisk can be used to mix everything to a smooth purée, but if you're going to make a habit of going without anything more solid for breakfast, it would be well worth investing in an electric blender.

Having said all that, if you've time to eat a bowl of cereal you'll be giving your system some roughage to work on too – and keeping hunger pangs at bay just that little longer. Most of the cereals you can buy in supermarkets are saturated with white sugar, though by no means all of them are. Again, the power of public pressure has been proven by the fact that an increasing number of manufacturers are reducing the amount of sugar they add to their products, especially if these are the kind considered to be 'healthy', such as varieties of muesli and crunchy oat-type cereals. Unfortunately, most of the cereals aimed specifically at children still seem to be over-sweetened, presumably on the assumption that children will turn their noses up at them if they're not.

Choose your cereal carefully. You can also easily make your own. For muesli all you need do is put a large bag of flaked mixed grains into a bowl, stir in nuts, desiccated coconut, dried fruit, whatever else takes your fancy. Store it in a jar or sealed polythene bag, add milk just before you're ready to eat (you can leave muesli to soak in milk overnight if you prefer, or even add just water which will still make the muesli creamy). Add fresh fruit if you like. Together with a glass of juice you'll have a well-balanced breakfast that takes no time to prepare, little more to eat.

If busy dieters are renowned for breakfasting on black coffee, their favourite lunch is invariably an apple and a chunk of cheese. They could do worse, but they could also do better.

Bread – a dirty word

It was back in the sixties that bread became a dirty word. Fashionable diets at that time were based on grapefruit, steaks and salad. Over recent years bread has come back into fashion, though it has changed somewhat – or rather, it's gone back to what it was way before the sixties. Wholemeal bread contains the bran most of us now know provides roughage, but in its natural form and – more important – a balanced amount. The mania for adding bran to everything very often did more harm than good; to a system unused to it, large amounts of bran can be uncomfortable if not positively dangerous! Wheat germ, rich in vitamin E, is another constituent of wholemeal bread. An average slice will contain approximately seventy calories,which is about the same as the apple and considerably less than even a small piece of cheese. And because the energy from grains is released slowly, you won't feel hungry during the afternoon either.

Which means that the quickest snack lunch – the sandwich – can also be surprisingly wholesome too. If you've time, make your own using lots of salad and just a small amount of protein. Cheese may be a favourite sandwich ingredient, egg a close second, but don't forget about nut butters, tahini, the many bean pâtés and spreads you can now buy ready-made at your local wholefood shop.

Too rushed to make your own? There are sandwich bars on most streets nowadays, as well as in food stores, bakers and department stores. If they don't already offer wholemeal bread, ask them. The same if you buy from a works canteen or office snack bar. Suggest the kind of fillings you'd like if they're not already on their menu. Show them there's a demand for real food and you'll encourage them to supply it. And if you can persuade them to offer a selection of fresh fruit at the same time – which many of them already do – you'll be able to pick up a quick snack that will keep you going all afternoon and longer.

The salad bar

A recent innovation in snack foods is that of salad bars where up to twenty or more different kinds of salad are displayed. You choose a small, medium or large container, fill it with the varieties of your choice, and pay a set price. Though the intention is good, and many of the salads *are* fresh, do think before you reach for the spoon if this kind of lunch appeals to you. Like everything in the food retail business, these salad bars are intended to be profitable. That means waste must be kept to a minimum, and that in turn means many of the varieties may well contain additives including preservatives. To be fair, some of the more reputable bars do have notices giving you the exact contents of each of the salads, and that includes additives. Many however do not. Bars with slow turnovers may also put out the same salad for more than a day, which could result in it not only being stale, but also full of bacteria. Remember, these salads are usually displayed uncovered and at room temperature. They may well be refrigerated overnight, but the changes from cold to warm then cold again can allow germs to remain undetected for longer.

By all means support these bars. They are ideal for anyone who enjoys salad but has little time to prepare it. But try to buy from establishments that are well used and therefore have a quick turnover, and check any labels if you're unsure whether or not a salad has preservatives in it or ask if there are no labels to check – and maybe suggest they correct this so they won't have to keep on answering other people? And learn to judge the freshness of a salad by its appearance. Food that's past its best has no place in your new way of eating.

So you've got through the day – it's dinner time and you're tired and hungry. What now?

Giving the little woman something to do

It was after the last war that the fashion began for cooking complicated dishes. Suddenly women had more time on their hands, magazines were full of new and challenging recipes, and when eventually rationing stopped, there was no excuse not to spend whole afternoons fiddling around in the kitchen. If not whole days!

Nowadays, though cooking the occasional special meal is still considered an enjoyable challenge by many, most women have other things to do with their time. They work, they study, they play sports, they go to the opera, they bring up families. Yet still they tend to feel guilty about not spending more time in the kitchen. It's as though the longer you take to prepare a meal, the more you must care.

Whether or not you choose to subscribe to that theory is up to you. You could, of course, put it the other way round. Because your time is precious, certainly equal in value to anyone else's, you owe it to yourself to spend as much time as you like in the kitchen – or as little.

Like other kinds of cuisines, wholefood cookery can be esoteric, sophisticated, requiring a pinch of this, a soupçon of that. But if you're not into pinches and soupçons, you can prepare many delicious meals in half the time and with the minimum of fuss. And if the general consensus of opinion seems to be that wholefood cookery takes forever, that's probably based on just one thing: beans. The pulses do need to be cooked slowly and for an hour or two, it's true. But it's easy enough to get them started, and then you can go away and forget them. In a slow cooker they'll simmer overnight or whilst you're out at work. Or use a pressure cooker and cut the time by at least half. You can also cook up far more than you need and keep them in the fridge to use within the next week, or the freezer where they can stay until you need them.

Besides, beans are only one ingredient. Other 'convenience' foods are tofu, bulgar, couscous, pasta, nuts, split lentils, plus dairy produce such as eggs, cheese, yogurt, all of which require the absolute minimum of cooking. Vegetables too are tastier and more nutritious when just lightly cooked. If time is a problem for you, forget about the more complicated dishes, at least whilst you're getting used to cooking with wholefoods. Build up a list of quick dishes you can put together in next to no time. Such a list might include pasta with a tofu tomato sauce, quick lentil curry, cauliflower with tahini sauce. Don't feel guilty about it. You can get around to the lasagnes, the pancakes, the stuffed mushrooms later, when you're used to the ingredients and when you have more time. Most important of all, when you *want* to.

On the subject of convenience foods, there are now a number of ranges of frozen foods that cater for people who want to eat only the best. These are usually made without any additives, the ingredients are either vegetarian or vegan, and some of them are also completely organic. Though I am not suggesting you rely on such foods all the time, they certainly have a valid role to play in a society where the value of eating good food is becoming more widely appreciated each day, and yet the pace of life makes it impossible to spend a lot of time preparing such foods.

Coping when you hate to cook

Hate cooking? You're not alone. The assumption that all women are at their happiest when pottering in the kitchen has probably got around because – until fairly recently – those that hated it were reluctant to admit as much. This goes back to the days when a woman's place was in the home, her role that of wife, mother, housekeeper and cook. Things have changed. Now you can be honest. But if that means you tend to live on take-aways, stop and think. How nutritious are they? Or just as important, how harmful? Chinese and Indian are the most popular, and such foods can of course be very good. But when they're cooked in bulk and kept warm until ordered or re-heated in a microwave, a lot of the vitamins and minerals will have been lost. So will the flavour.

Have the occasional take-away if you must, but aim to eat mostly food you've bought and prepared yourself. It doesn't have to be complicated. Live on soup, toast and peanut butter – you could do a lot worse. Eat more raw foods which many nutritionalists say is the healthiest way to eat anyway. Or go for simple dishes like the ones listed above, none of which takes long to prepare, and most of which have little or no chance of going wrong. Use them even when entertaining, if you like. They can be spruced up for guests by the addition of just one expensive and unusual ingredient: a sprinkling of pistachios over the bulgar pilaf, wild rice with the curry, tiny out-of-season new potatoes with the cauliflower. Don't think that you have to like cooking in order to change to eating the wholefood way. You don't. You don't even have to like eating very much – though you may well find your attitude changes once you get a taste of what food should really taste like.

The business lunch

Maybe your job is the kind that has you attending high-powered business lunches every so often, possibly very often. Once upon a time that might have put pay to any healthy eating plan, but nowadays it needn't. To start with vegetarian restaurants are springing up all over the place, and very good some of them are too. If you don't have one nearby, most reasonable restaurants include at least one vegetarian dish on the menu (even Berni Steak Houses do!). There is more emphasis on vegetables and salads than there ever used to be and desserts usually include fresh fruit. Of course, there are still many restauranteurs whose idea of a salad is a spoonful of coleslaw and a slice of pickled beetroot. If you have any say – and if you're taking a client out you have the choice, and if you're the guest your opinion surely matters? – avoid such places.

Alcohol is often an important part of business lunches. The same with parties and all sorts of social occasions. We're told that the British as a people drink too much, and that alcohol contributes to a wide range of illnesses – not to mention accidents on the road. We're advised to restrict ourselves to no more than fourteen units per week for a woman, twenty-one for a man. A unit is one small glass of wine, a single measure of spirits, a half pint of beer. And yet we rely increasingly on alcohol to have a good time, to give ourselves courage, to cheer ourselves.

One major disadvantage is that most alcoholic drinks are high in calories and virtually devoid of nutrients. What's more, the calories are used straight away which means that others – from food, for example – are stored. On the plus side, there is a theory that says a small amount of good quality wine helps strengthen the immune system, and we all know it can work wonders when we are tense.

Even if you enjoy drinking, the business lunch is one occasion when you need to keep a clear head. Yet it's difficult to say no without appearing to be a spoilsport, an outsider. What should you do?

There is no right answer to this dilemma, but there's an answer for *you*. Again, think about it, make up your mind and then stick to your decision. You can just enjoy the wine and not worry (if you're eating at the same time the food will of course help you stay relatively sober). Or have just one glass and make it last. Or water it down with still mineral water. Or say you don't drink. If you genuinely do need an excuse, mumble something about your doctor! Keeping your alcohol consumption under control isn't easy because after a few glasses your control tends to go out of the window, but as with everything in life, the choice is yours. If after careful consideration you decide a certain amount of alcohol won't harm you, and that you know what you're doing, then carry on drinking. If however you make up your mind to cut back, even to stop drinking, you can do it. A diet full of vitamins and minerals will help you in either case so don't feel – as some people do – that because you can't correct every single aspect of your life at one go, you might as well give up altogether!

House-bound and hungry

Being at home all day can create a whole variety of different problems. If you're busy you'll probably be disinclined to prepare proper food for yourself, skipping lunch, keeping yourself going on coffee and biscuits. Boredom can lead to much the same habit. If you've got young children around you may well find yourself picking at the bits they don't want. It's this way of eating that has many young house-bound mums putting on weight and wondering why. Yet they may never really enjoy their food, partly because they're not aware of what's going into their mouths – but also, who can enjoy a diet of other people's left-overs?

If you are eating badly out of boredom you've got no excuse.

Use those empty hours to clean out the cupboard and fridge and re-stock with wholesome foods. No reason why you shouldn't still eat biscuits, cakes, whatever you like, but make sure they have something to offer besides a sweet taste – better still, make them yourself. Learning to cook with natural ingredients can be fun, so can producing some of those ingredients yourself. Try sprouting beans or wholegrains, growing herbs, making bread. And if the thought of cooking bores you – get out of the house and do something else! Nowadays there are classes on just about everything, sports to try, people needing company, so many things you can do to take your mind off having nothing to do!

Being trapped in a house with young children doesn't mean you can't also make changes in the way you eat. Instead of setting yourself apart from the rest of the family, though, include them in your new approach to food. Children in particular will benefit from having eaten wholefoods from early in life. Allergies, hyperactivity, a tendency to catch every bug that is going; these and other childhood problems can be improved if not completely cured by a change of diet. Never say 'This is good for you'. Or 'Eat this, and afterwards you can have a sweet'. Turn things round the other way. For example, a dried fruit bar could replace the sweet. They're easy to make, cost less than the manufactured variety – and you'll know exactly what's in them. Even better, get your children to help in the kitchen. Things might be a little chaotic, but they'll learn far more about food and nutrition from getting their fingers in the bowl than from having their noses in books!

Whilst they're learning, of course, you'll be learning with them. It will be a shared experience, which is one of the best ways to do things. Just remember not to let it become a chore. Children are especially sensitive to moods and if you're not enjoying yourself, neither will they.

Living on peanuts

If there's one section of society that has taken to vegetarianism and wholefoods in a big way over recent years, it's those in their late teens and early twenties, females in particular. Mostly this is because of concern about the cruelty involved with the production of animal foods, but along with it goes an encouraging awareness of the importance of eating natural foods. Many of these converts are students, or just starting out in careers, or maybe even unemployed – and when money is tight, the housekeeping is the first thing to be cut. The expression 'living on peanuts' can take on a whole new meaning!

Wholefoods are generally not expensive, especially when compared with meat and fish. Wholegrains and pulses are especially good value for money. But a varied diet is important, and that means including as many different ingredients as possible. Free-range eggs are without doubt preferable to those that come from factory farms, but they can cost twice as much if not more. Wholemeal bread is usually more expensive than the refined white variety that is sold in such bulk that manufacturers can cut the cost and still be in pocket. Most nuts are high in price, crops being affected by all sorts of problems, and their collection and removal from shells being labour intensive. Organic vegetables are still only grown on a small scale in Britain, the bulk of government subsidies going to those who use chemicals despite growing public demand for vegetables grown without them. This means the price of organically grown produce can be anything from expensive to exorbitant.

The answer is to base your diet on the cheap foods and use the more expensive items as garnishes. This is how the majority of the British used meat a century or so ago; their main dish was based on cereals, pulses, vegetables, and just a little meat was added to give extra flavour and nutrition. In fact, it's only since we could afford to eat meat at least once a day, and in huge slabs rather than using it as a garnish, that we have become such an unhealthy nation. Instead of meat use nuts, seeds, tofu, a little dairy produce to add extra protein with the minimum of saturated fats.

If you're living on a very limited budget, chances are you also have only minimal space in which to prepare and cook your food. Organisation is the key here. Use wall space for storage, buy stacking jars and saucepans, hang the equipment you use most often – knives, whisks and so on – from hooks on a peg board. Keep everything to the minimum. Especially useful are a small coffee grinder (use it for nuts too), a fold-up stainless steel steamer that will fit in any saucepan, kitchen scissors, whisk, a good knife and a wooden spoon. You'll be surprised how many dishes you can produce with just these few items. Later, when you've money and space, you can add to them.

Whatever your problem, there are ways to overcome it. Don't let anything put you off eating the wholefood way.

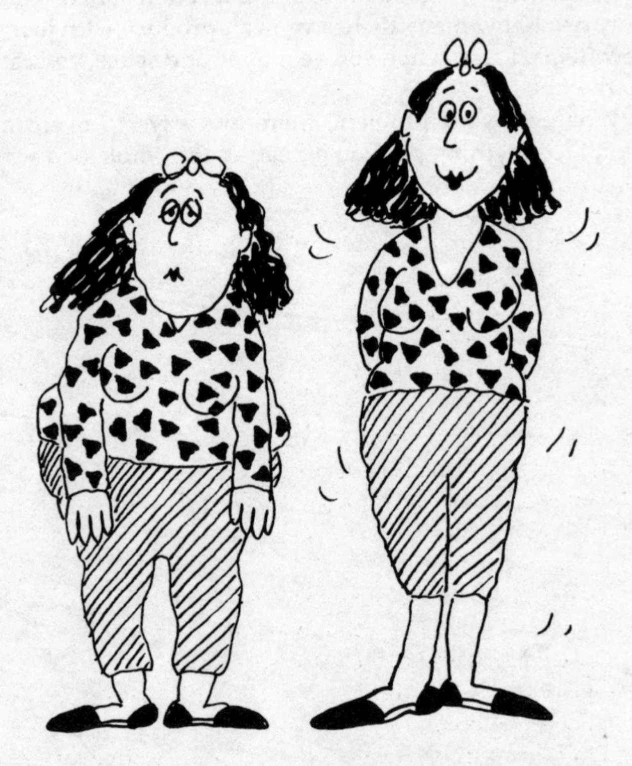

By standing straight you will reduce your spare tyre

5 *F*at feelings

QUIZ

1 Do you sometimes *feel* especially fat even when your scales indicate that you haven't put on any weight?
2 Is just before a period one of the times when you suffer from fat feelings?
3 Do you tend to eat next to nothing during the day, make up for it at night?
4 If you usually have your main meal in the evening, at what time do you sit down to eat?
5 Do you ever eat when you are tense and/or angry?
6 If so, how does this affect your enjoyment of the meal?
7 Do you ever suffer from indigestion?
8 If so, what do you think causes it?
   a) the foods eaten?
   b) the speed at which you ate?
   c) your state of mind at the time?
   d) some physical cause?
9 Do you ever get vague aches, especially in your back, neck and shoulders?
10 Do you find you feel tired much of the time, even when there is no obvious reason?

Faulty scales?

Fat feelings don't necessarily have anything to do with being fat. You can get them even when your scales confirm you haven't put on a pound – you might even have lost weight since you last checked. And they're very reliable scales!

So why do you still feel bloated, uncomfortable, as though you've just eaten a five course meal? Fat feelings can have a vareity of different causes, most of which you can do something about. First, though, you need to analyse which of them applies to you.

For women in their child-bearing years, water retention just before a period is a common problem. Its effects – though temporary – are very real. You may find you feel tender all over, sore, your waist may seem to expand (and it can in fact be an inch or two larger). Water pressure around the brain is what gives you mood swings. Though you won't necessarily weigh more than usual, some women do gain anything up to seven pounds. Half our body weight is made up of water – about seventy pints – a complicated system keeping this amount steady. It is a hormone imbalance, often caused by nutritional deficiencies, that makes the kidneys less efficient at doing their job. There are a number of steps you can take to lessen these effects. Diuretic herbal tablets will help; buy them in a combination specially chosen to be gently effective. Hot herb teas can also be of some use – especially good is chamomile which is a diuretic and also a relaxant. Many women find homeopathic medicines a positive help; others swear by vitamin B6 supplements which they claim relieve some if not all of the symptoms.

The food you eat can also help alleviate water retention. Bitter foods such as raddichio and watercress will stimulate the liver and pancreas, thus helping them get your water content back into balance. Trials in Toronto, Canada (reported in *The Lancet* in 1989) indicated that by reducing fats to a minimum and increasing starchy foods, nine out of ten premenstrual women were helped, many of them saying the heavy feeling was lessened, their breasts not so painful. As carbohydrates are also useful in helping to steady a low blood sugar level – something else many women suffer from just before a period, which is what has them rushing for the chocolates! – you could do worse than boost your grain consumption for a week or so each month. That doesn't mean you have to live on bowls of barley (though do, by all means, if you enjoy it). Wholegrain breads are ideal, and consider the many crackers and crispbreads now available, some made with rye, others with oats or rice.

Cutting back on salt

Salt, of course, is a major contributor to the problem of water retention. If you suffer this way, cut back your salt intake at all times, but especially just before a period. Don't use it in your cooking at all – use herbs and pepper to flavour food instead. Look out too for ingredients that come ready salted. Crisps, peanuts and soya sauce are obvious, but there's salt hidden away in more processed and convenience foods than you may realise. If you must eat such foods, check the labels. An excessive craving for salt can indicate that the mineral salt content in your body is out of balance – if you must, use rock salt or low sodium salt, both of which contain essential minerals such as iodine and potassium, but still keep it to a minimum.

It is also wise to cut out or at least reduce your consumption of alcohol at that time. Because the body tissues retain more water, any alcohol will stay in the body longer than usual making the effects also last longer, and feel stronger. Constipation is another problem often associated with that week or so before a period. It also, of course, affects both women and men at all other stages of their lives, though it is especially prevalent in the elderly who may well eat less and – because of less-than-efficient teeth and digestive systems – often prefer refined foods. Over recent years the harm constipation can cause to health has been well highlighted. It can also, of course, make you feel full and swollen.

Though the wonders of bran have been extolled not just via the media, but also by the medical profession, adding bran to a diet based on refined and processed food is entirely the wrong way to approach this problem. It's rather like being on a diet, ordering a huge chocolate sundae topped with fudge sauce and cream – and then insisting on a low calorie wafer to dip into it! Bran is the fibrous part of a grain (usually wheat or oat) that has been extracted during the process of making flour or flakes. Certainly bran will help keep your system functioning regularly. A far better way, however, is to obtain your fibre direct from source where it occurs in balance with other nutrients. Wholefoods are just that – *whole* foods. If in their natural form they contain fibre, they will reach your table with most of that fibre intact. Eat such foods every day and constipation will no longer be a problem. A point to remember: as wholemeal flour contains phytic acid which can block the absorption of some minerals, calcium in particular, aim to vary the grains you eat. Oats are especially good and are now widely recommended to help reduce cholesterol build-up.

All in the mind

The link between our minds and bodies has already been mentioned. How we think very much affects our choice of food, our way of eating, and the pleasure we derive from it. We can also use our minds not only to understand the psychological and physical importance of food in our lives – but to control and even to change this. Making up our minds; isn't that the expression?

Though we sometimes forget it, ultimately our minds are all-powerful.

If, then, we sit down to eat whilst our heads are spinning, chances are our bodies will be affected. To be really enjoyed, a meal should be eaten in a relaxed frame of mind. We should take time to notice what we are eating, to savour the separate tastes, to listen for that inner voice that says stop, you've had enough.

Unfortunately, eating is rarely this kind of experience. If you are eating socially, with friends or family, conversation may be stimulating, amusing, even heated. Business lunches require you to be aware of what you're saying, maybe even to make important decisions. However much at ease you might appear to be, you're alert. The adrenalin is flowing.

Even snack meals are invariably hurried meals squeezed in between one o'clock and two, or between one activity and the next. Nowadays, many of them are actually eaten whilst you're standing, maybe whilst you're on the move.

Is it any wonder that every day literally millions of people end up taking tablets for indigestion?

Indigestion can cause anything from mild stomach pains, wind, a feeling of being pumped up, to cramps, heartburn and even severe spasms in the upper chest that can be mistaken for angina or a heart attack. Most certainly it can make you feel fat. It can also cause sleeplessness, irritability, and in chronic cases can affect your general health, your work and home life. Surprising, then, how lightly it is taken. Most people think of it as an inconvenience rather than an illness, something they just have to learn to live with.

So you think your digestive system is not coping as well as it ought with the food you eat? In rare cases this can be because of a physical malfunction such as a hiatus hernia or ulcers. Anyone who suffers from chronic indigestion over a long period, and for no obvious reason, would be wise to check with a doctor. Most likely, though, your indigestion is a result of your life style or your eating habits – or both. If that's the case, you can almost certainly do something about it.

Some foods are known to be more difficult to digest than others. Chocolate causes problems, so do acidy ingredients such as vinegar. Best known though are fatty meats, beans, watercress and onions. To an extent this can be overcome by the way in which these ingredients are cooked and served. Traditional dishes include herbs – sage and mint, for example, help your body digest fat. Apple sauce is another favourite. Yogurt is served with curries and spicy Middle Eastern dishes, smooth and creamy hummus with felafels.

Spot the villains

If you can identify certain ingredients that are troublesome to your digestive system, the obvious thing to do is try to avoid them. Unless they are the mainstay of a meal, you can usually push them to the side of your plate. Another trick when you're dining out is to eat some bread at the same time; this helps bind the troublemaker and ease its passage. Make sure though that you chew the bread well, especially if it is wholemeal.

There are some foods, however, that form an integral part of the wholefood diet, and if you learn how to make them more acceptable you can only benefit. All pulses contain substances in the skin that hinder the digestive process and can cause flatulence; a few contain toxins when raw. The smaller varieties such as lentils obviously cook quicker and more thoroughly. Look out too for those now available in the form of flakes – soya flakes are especially easy to use and just as nutritious as the whole beans (which can take up to three hours to cook, or even longer if they're not too fresh!). Even with the larger beans, however, you can prevent problems by making sure you cook them properly. Start by soaking them in cold water, preferably overnight. Or when time is limited, cover them with boiling water and leave for an hour instead. Though some experts recommend cooking the beans in the soaking water (this does help retain some of the nutrients), they are without doubt more easily digested if rinsed thoroughly and then cooked in fresh water. Don't add salt either – this toughens the skin. First boil them for 10 minutes, then simmer until tender. When ready, use them in the recipe of your choice, preferably flavouring them with herbs and balancing them with other ingredients – even the strongest digestive system is going to be unable to cope with a large plate of nothing but beans! And if you're not used to eating pulses, do introduce them gradually to your diet to enable your stomach to adjust.

Watercress is an excellent salad ingredient, rich in iron and with a distinctive peppery taste. If you find it hard to eat raw, put it into a sandwich, or make a soup or soufflé with it. Raw onions can be used in a salad if you chop them fine and keep them to a minimum; a yogurt dressing would be an ideal aid to digestion. Experiment with other ingredients in much the same way. You may well find yourself enjoying something you used to think you hated! If not, though, don't force yourself to eat it. Remember that an important aspect of this new way of eating is that it should always be a pleasurable experience.

Finish your meal with a cup of herb tea – apart from the obvious peppermint and fennel, try lemon balm which is lovely and fresh tasting as well as being excellent for your digestion.

Social eating is, of course, a popular pastime in much of the Western world. Statistics indicate that we in Britain dine out more often than we ever used to, that restaurants and other eating establishments are on the increase, as are their profits. And when we're not paying to eat out we're being invited to dine with friends, or having them round to join us. Cordon Bleu cookery has reached the masses with everyone tucking into dishes with French names and rich sauces, into desserts that are works of art in sugar and cream.

Overeating is another cause of indigestion. It isn't that any of the foods particularly disagree with us – just that there's too much there for our stomachs to work on. Very often we go straight to bed which makes matters worse.

Is food more fattening if eaten as a large meal at night? Some experts believe there is an element of truth in this. The body's metabolic rate speeds up and burns calories at a faster rate after a meal, and if you are active at the same time it will do so more effectively. However, this does appear to differ from person to person. Certainly though, a large meal eaten late at night will do nothing to give you a sound night's sleep. A good general policy would be to try to spread your daily food intake more evenly through the day, and to eat no later than seven except on those special occasions.

Taut as a violin string

Also try to avoid eating meals when tense or over-tired. Not only will your body not be in a fit state to digest your food properly, but you'll actually be putting more of a strain on it.

By all means have a light snack, or a drink such as one made with tofu, milk or yogurt whisked together with fruit juice. Then relax, rest, and forget about eating for a while. Indigestion is just one of the problems that comes with tension – and it may even be one of the least serious. Others include raised blood pressure, heart trouble, depression. If you have a tendency to go around feeling about as taut as a violin string, maybe you should do something about it? There are many techniques currently being taught to help, some based on taking more physical exercise, others helping you slow down your whole system, to unwind, to get back in touch again with your true self. Do explore such things as meditation, biofeedback, yoga. Treat yourself to a course of massage treatments. Most important of all, make a point of allowing yourself some time each day in which to do absolutely nothing. It's a strange paradox: you can improve your digestion, your health, your quality of life by doing nothing. It could even *save* your life.

Waist not, want not

Statistically, the British female has a tendency towards being pear shaped, with hips and thighs causing most concern. Just the same, it's around your waist that you probably first notice any weight loss – or gain. Strange thing is, you may find yourself feeling fat around the waist even when you haven't put on weight. Call it what you like: a spare tyre, midriff bulge. Either way it's uncomfortable, it puts a strain on zips, it ruins the way your clothes hang. As it so often seems to happen in women in their middle years, some people call it Middle Age Spread, and it's easy to see why. But there is also a clue here.

Convinced you have the start of a spare tyre – or even a well-established one? Try this. Stand up, feet together, arms loose at your sides, back straight. Now try to stand taller, lifting from the back of your head as though someone has attached a piece of string to a strand of hair. Feel your upper body pulling up away from your hips.

Though your tyre may not have gone, it's sure to be less

obvious. Pull in your stomach and it will improve a little more. In other words, by working on your posture you may be able to eliminate your spare tyre altogether.

But slumping – you may say – is a natural part of the ageing process, our bodies curling like autumn leaves. And it's true that the average sixty-five year old will be some five centimetres (nearly two inches) shorter than she or he was at twenty. It's all to do with muscle tone, elasticity, the fact that most of us become less active, give up sports, take the car or bus instead of walking. It may well be natural, but it isn't always inevitable. Think of ballet dancers. Their super-awareness of how they hold themselves and the way they move is obvious, even when they're not dancing. Many of them remain involved with the ballet for all their lives, even into old age, maybe teaching or becoming choreographers. It is rare to find a single spare tyre amongst them.

Think of those films we often see on television these days showing primitive tribes, people living simple lives close to nature. How often they include elderly women carrying water on their heads, their walk graceful, each step confident, their spines straight. Their lives may be hard. But the fact that they must rely on their bodies for so much means that they remain healthy and strong considerably longer than those in the same age group in the affluent countries of the West.

Of course, if you're young you have no excuse for those extra inches around the waist. Bad posture will eventually cause you far more problems than a spare tyre. Rounded shoulders will lead to aches in your back and neck. A contracted rib cage will lessen the efficiency of your lungs so that you take shallow breaths, don't get as much oxygen as you should. Your digestive organs won't be able to work properly. Because your body will be out of alignment, walking and carrying things will become more difficult and therefore more tiring. If your spine is distorted, you may eventually need to walk with a stick.

All this because of bad posture? It's possible.

What is certain is that by standing straight you will reduce your spare tyre. You'll also be putting across a whole different message about yourself to the world. You'll be saying that you're happy to meet people, to face things as they are, that you enjoy challenges. You'll be saying you like yourself too, which is a good positive way to approach life. It also tends to make other people feel much the same way.

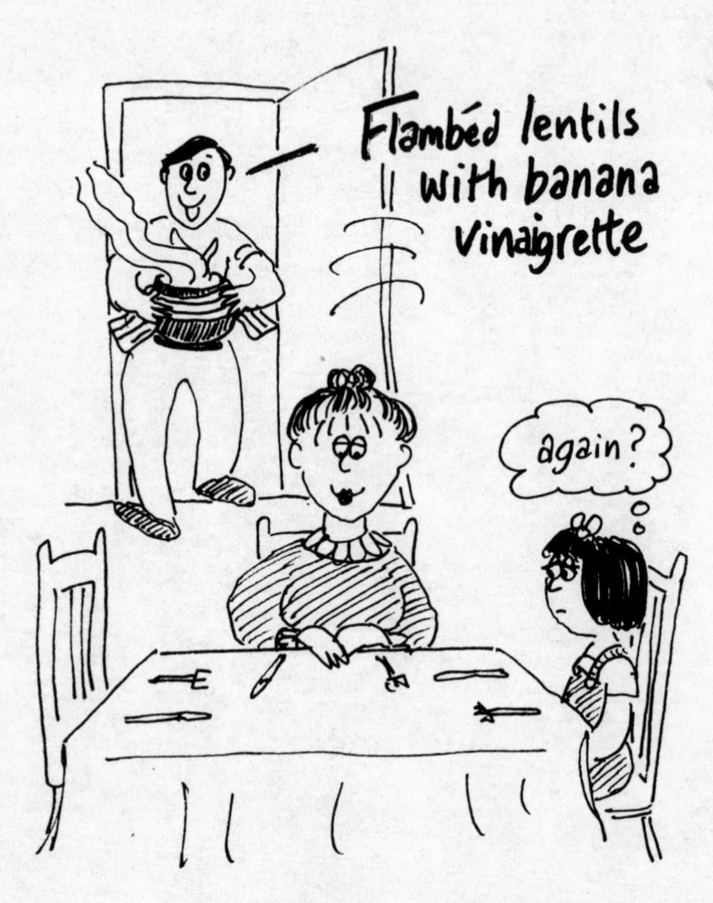

Why not take it in turns to cook?

6 *M*an in the kitchen

QUIZ

1 Is the man in your life concerned about eating healthily?
2 Does he consider himself to be overweight? Do you?
3 If he does, what is it that most worries him?
  a) his appearance?
  b) an increased chance of illness?
  c) increased insurance premiums?
4 What is the most likely reason for this extra weight?
5 Would he be prepared to take the responsibility for doing anything about it?
6 When eating at home, do you prepare his meals?
7 If he also cooks, is this because
  a) he feels obliged to take his turn?
  b) you insist he does so?
  c) he enjoys it?
8 What is his favourite type of food?
  a) good old fashioned stodge?
  b) steak?
  c) salads, vegetables and fruit?
9 Does he eat out
  a) every day?
  b) once a week?
  c) only rarely?
10 If he drinks alcohol regularly, what does he prefer?
  a) beer?
  b) wine?
  c) spirits?

Men lag behind

In a recent Mori poll, men were questioned about their attitudes to food in general and healthy eating in particular. Their answers will probably come as no surprise to most women. They indicated that men lagged well behind women when it came to any willingness to change the way they ate; in fact, many of those who said they had taken on board at least some of the latest ideas (cutting saturated fats, eating more fibre) admitted that they'd virtually been coerced to do so when their wives had changed their own eating habits. Those who had done so willingly had usually become aware of the need only after they themselves, or someone close to them, had become ill.

Why is this? And can anything be done to encourage men to care more about themselves and their health *before* those first symptoms appear to indicate that something is already going wrong?

In a society where a woman feels she must look attractive if she is to be accepted, successful, loved and ultimately happy, men need other qualities. Even as boys they have less body awareness, are rarely encouraged to seek approval for looks alone. A proud mum might boast of her pretty daughter, but she'll be more likely to tell how well her son is doing at school, or what a great sense of humour he has, or how he's been picked for the cricket team.

Despite this, many boys do become suddenly aware of their looks in their teens, often dressing in a conspicuous way to show that they belong with their own generation, and have absolutely nothing whatsoever to do with the rest of us! Once they were Mods and Rockers, more recently they've been Punks. The majority of them grow out of this phase and develop the attitude so typical of British men, one that puts clothes and appearance low on their list of priorities.

To some extent men *have* become more aware of their looks over recent years. Now there are seasonal fashions for men, as for women. Men spend more money than ever before on haircuts, colognes and after shaves. It's no longer considered effeminate for a man to care about the way he looks, or how he smells, or even how he feels. Many of the trendy young men about town do eat healthy foods; they also work out in a gym or go jogging each day before breakfast, watch their alcohol intake, will extol the benefits of Royal Jelly and ginseng.

A trendy minority

Such men are, however, a trendy and mostly well-heeled minority. And amongst them there are many who are motivated, encouraged or cajoled by the women in their lives. At the other end of the spectrum there are those stalwarts who refuse to give up foods they've eaten all their lives, who wouldn't dream of walking when they can drive, who think a few extra pounds (or stones!) make a man more of a man. Tell them that they'll probably live longer if they change their ways, and they'll shrug it off or even laugh in your face. Tell them that they'll feel better from day to day, have more energy, sleep more soundly, and they'll say they're doing fine as they are, thanks very much. If stubbornness was an indication of masculinity, these men would be the Rambos of the neighbourhood!

Trouble is, they're doing themselves no favours. Reluctant as they might be, they would certainly feel better for changing their way of eating. They may well look better too. Even more important, statistics show that they'll increase their chances of living to a ripe old age.

Britain is one of the world leaders in death from coronary heart disease with 5,000 deaths each week, the majority of them men between the ages of thirty and sixty. Deaths from cancer are also horrifyingly high. It's well known that diet, along with smoking, is a major contributory factor in both these diseases. Many of these premature deaths, if not the majority, can be avoided, but only if action is taken early, if changes are made. If the resolution to live a full and long life is accompanied not by crossed fingers, but by a positive health plan.

So why is it that the majority of men seem reluctant to make such changes?

Food, in our society, is deemed the responsibility of women. The kitchen is where food is prepared. Therefore, from an early age most males are taught not to interfere or get in the way, or better still, to stay out of the kitchen altogether. By feeding her family, a mother shows she cares. She also has a unique role in home life, a room that is her territory and into which others can come only if she agrees. Not only does this instil in any male children that kitchens are forbidden places and nothing to do with them, but on a more practical level it means they never learn how to do anything even as simple as boiling an egg!

If in later years they marry – as probably most of them will – their wives or girlfriends take over this role. Inevitably, because she does the cooking the woman also decides exactly what she is going to cook, which ingredients she will use and where she will buy them. This, after all, is what women in our society are taught to do. She will also decide how nutritious or otherwise the meals she serves will be, which means her man can be literally putting his life in her hands.

If this sound like a description of your man, and should you both be perfectly happy for things to continue as they are, there is nothing more to be said. If, however, you would prefer him to take at least some responsibility for his own health, you have a challenge ahead. What you need to do first is encourage him to think about how he eats and to decide if there is anything he can do to improve it.

Is he always tired?

His general health is an indication of the quality of the food he eats. Is he always tired, lacking the enthusiasm to try something new, go somewhere different? How does he sleep? Can he relax without needing a Scotch or two to help him? Is he sometimes edgy, moody?

How he looks can also tell him a lot about what's going on inside. Eyes are an instant giveaway, so is skin. So, of course, is body weight. If he's very thin it might be that he's not eating enough, or that his body isn't absorbing the nutrients from the food he consumes, maybe because of a vitamin or mineral imbalance caused by stress or over-tiredness. Even if he is overweight – and when you consider how sedentary are the lives of most businessmen, it isn't surprising to find that many of them are – it could well be that he is under-nourished.

Though the woman who thinks she is overweight has her doubts continually reinforced by clothing manufacturers who seem to consider fashions can only be worn by skinnies, by the media pushing the Slim is In message, and by Page Three girls daring to reveal all because there isn't that much to reveal, men have none of these reminders. Even severely overweight men have a wide choice of not just sizes but styles when they shop for clothing. You only have to read the advertisements for new slimming products to see that their target market is women; how often do they feature a man jumping for joy in a bikini? And the Page Three boy is not yet a regular, at least not with any of the national newspapers.

No wonder then that men in general are so unconcerned about their shape. And why should they be? If your man is just a little overweight but feels fit (and can afford to buy a new shirt when the buttons won't do up on the old one!) the last thing he'll want or even need to do is diet.

Just the same, excess weight is usually caused by eating too many foods that are high in fat and calories but low in nutrition. In other words, unhealthy food. His weight could be an indication that he needs to look at the kind of things he's eating, not just at home but during the day when he may be working in a factory or office, or out on the road.

Because most men go out to work, they will eat at least five meals away from home each week. Business lunches may be an important part of his job, so may the drinking of alcohol. He may have no choice but to eat at transport cafes or works canteens where the menu is based on the traditional combination of stodge, fats and tomato ketchup. Many men get into the habit of hardly eating during the day, living off coffees and their nerves instead, then make up for it by gorging in the evening.

All of this is out of your control, of course. But it isn't out of *his*. Only he can decide how much his health matters to him and – if he considers it important enough – can make at least some changes. Choose more appropriate dishes from restaurant menus, avoid places that offer no appropriate dishes at all. Take packed lunches if that's the only way to ensure he gets something worth eating.

Men more prone to some illness

Any man who has stopped and thought about how he eats is off to a good start. If he's the kind who likes to know the facts, get him to read one of the many excellent books on healthy eating. All the things that apply to your eating habits also apply to his, though men are more prone to certain illnesses. Along with stress and smoking, cholesterol is suspected of being a major factor in heart disease. Most of it is found in saturated fats. A third of the saturated fat in our diet comes from meat (along with a host of other dubious additives), so it makes sense to cut down on meat – or cut it out altogether. Dairy products are another source, and though they add not just protein but variety to a meal, he should try to keep them to a minimum. Instead, suggest he eats whole and natural foods such as grains, pulses, nuts, vegetables and fruit, all of which are low in saturated fats and calories – and they're very filling too.

If you think the details would bore him, or even put him off altogether, what about a cookbook or two? It's surprising how many men harbour a secret yearning to cook and are only waiting to be invited to join you in the kitchen. And once they've found out what's what and where you hide the whisk, they often make excellent cooks. Maybe the fact that they've never considered cooking a duty might have something to do with it? What's more, most men are not inhibited by the training that tends to make women combine only those ingredients they've learned go well together, be thrifty, be cautious. A man in the kitchen will probably use every saucepan there is, and the washing up may well take him (or you!) the rest of the evening, but his meals will rarely be dull.

Encourage your man to share your kitchen and you might

even find you learn something from him about the adventure that is cookery!

Why not take it in turn to cook? Or work together, each doing different tasks? Get him to actually plan the menu sometimes too. *And* – if he has time – to do the shopping, at least now and again. Shopping is another of those jobs women accept as their privilege. Those who send their men to do it usually regret it, men tending to shop in the same extravagent manner as they cook! Yet preparing a meal starts with choosing ingredients, judging if they are fresh as well as value for money. Seeing what's available will also (hopefully) give him ideas for more meals.

Who says you have to be alone?

Ultimately, the aim is to make your man aware of food and the pleasure it can give – to prepare as well as to eat. Society may say a woman's place is in the kitchen, but it doesn't insist that she has to be alone.

Food isn't the only thing a man needs to watch out for. Though more women drink regularly now than ever before, and alcohol abuse amongst women is growing, it is still men who are more likely to drop in to the pub on the way home to unwind after a hectic day, or to get in the mood for an evening out, or to celebrate or cheer themselves up. Alcoholism is not only an illness in itself, it can lead to lack of confidence, problems at work and home, and ultimately to much worse. And because the effects on the body of drinking just a little too much can be slow to show up, the damage can be done before the danger is realised. Social drinking, providing it is under control, will do little harm. A man of average height and build can drink up to twenty-one units a week – but be sure he watches out for drinks such as extra strength lager that contain almost three times as much alcohol as ordinary lager!

Alcoholic sounds too strong a word? You're probably right. But do remember that an alcoholic isn't always a down-and-out who sleeps in the street and lives out of dustbins. Nor do alcoholics necessarily drink every day, nor start in the mornings, nor knock back slugs of neat vodka. The term applies to anyone who – once started – finds it impossible to stop drinking. They may only drink at weekends, even less frequently, they may never touch anything except beer or Babychams, but it is the compulsion to continue that indicates they have a problem. In time, such a problem can only damage their livers – not to mention their lives.

If your man is relying heavily on alcohol, try suggesting he cuts back a little or maybe drinks some of the excellent low alcohol brands that are now so widely available. Avoiding alcohol completely for a few days each week gives the body time to clean out the system, reduces the potential for damage. Should he be unable to do this, do persuade him to seek help – there are centres throughout the country. Go with him if that will help. Make the effort now, before it is too late.

Of course, changing the eating and drinking habits of a grown man will not be easy. In general, men do seem more wary of change. Maybe their determination to refuse to eat anything but the foods they've always eaten is a way of asserting themselves. Assertiveness shows strength and that a man must show he is strong is another of the attitudes dinned into many a boy. Like so many other things in today's world, that attitude too is fast changing. Often it shows more courage, more sense of adventure to let go of the past, to break away from the crowd, and start all over again.

If you are in the process of working through your own attitudes to food and your body, why not invite him to join you? Sharing and discovering together is fun. You can give encouragement when it's needed, know that there's someone there to back you should the going get a little difficult. And talking together will bring more dimensions to the subject, enable you to really begin to understand not just how food affects you – physically, emotionally and socially – but how it affects everyone.

A changed attitude to eating will gradually change your life. You'll feel fitter whilst at the same time finding yourself more relaxed about food, not worrying so much about what's in what, whether or not you should eat something, alternating between promising yourself rewards or punishments. In other words, you'll be free to *enjoy* your food. If the man in your life works with you the pleasure will be doubled.

Children and the seeds you sow

If you have children, you have a golden opportunity to set them on the right path from the beginning. You can encourage them to have a positive attitude to wholefoods whilst being confident that you're giving them the nutrients they need to grow strong, healthy and intelligent. It was, after all, in your early years and teens that most of your own attitudes to food were planted. Even nowadays women who should know better are encouraging their teenage daughters to diet when it is far from necessary. Theories for this vary. Do they subconsciously wish to stop them maturing into women, wanting to keep them skinny and childlike just a little bit longer? Are they aiming to prove they still have power over their daughters? Or is it to compensate for the fuller figures they may have and have still not come to accept? A vicarious way of enjoying all the supposed kudos and glamour of being skinny? Whatever the reason it is no excuse for setting their daughters on a pattern that may well stay with them – and haunt them! – for the rest of their lives.

Though some boys will have no more interest in food than wanting to know where the bread knife is, a surprising number will be more than happy to join in with the cooking, and from quite an early age. If your son show such a tendency, do encourage it. It's because society deems women to be in charge of food that boys who *have* any interest are sometimes reluctant to show it, worried that their schoolmates will think them cissy or effeminate, anticipating the teasing. Too often they are right. Trouble is, the myth then becomes self-perpetuating. Only when more mothers not only allow but actually encourage the whole family to join them in the kitchen will this attitude change. And as with all major social changes, it is the individuals who set them in motion. Individuals like you.

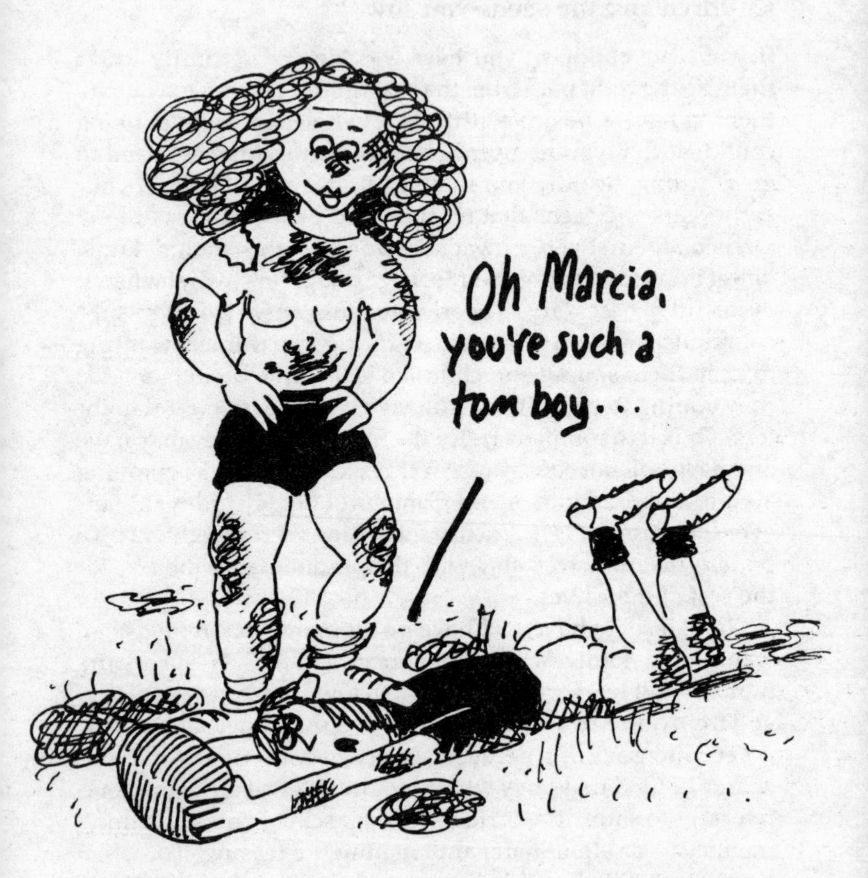

If you don't mind roughing it, how about taking up rugby?

7 The exercise factor

QUIZ

1 What do you think exercise can do for you?
   a) strengthen your heart?
   b) firm up your muscles?
   c) make you lose weight?
   d) change your mood?
   e) improve your sex life?
2 Do you have a car?
3 If so, do you use it
   a) every day?
   b) a couple of times a week?
   c) when going on long trips only?
4 How far do you walk on average each day?
   a) just around the house?
   b) at least a mile?
   c) further?
5 When faced with the choice between stairs and a lift, which do you usually opt for?
6 Did you enjoy playing games at school?
7 Or did you do whatever was necessary to get out of them?
8 Would you say you
   a) have a strong competitive urge?
   b) enjoy a challenge but have no great need to come first?
   c) are happiest when free from any pressures?
9 Have you ever attended an exercise class of any kind?
10 If so, but you gave it up, what made you decide to do so?

How to feel fully alive

Eating is just one aspect of the bid for good health. The other – without which no one can expect to feel really vital and fully alive – is exercise. Even though moving energetically will speed up the metabolism temporarily (you can tell by the fact that you feel hotter), few people will actually lose weight by exercise alone. If you've spent time studying calories you'll know that it takes about half an hour of walking to work off the calories from one medium slice of bread, whilst a more strenuous activity such as playing tennis for half an hour will only use up the calories from two such slices. The heavier you are, the more calories you are likely to use, though the difference is minimal. Should the scales show you *have* lost a pound or two, most likely it will be in perspiration and you'll put it back on again as soon as you have that drink you're craving. So why exercise? Because of the many far more important benefits it offers.

Start a regular routine, and within a very short time your muscle tone will improve, which will make you look slimmer and firmer even if your weight is exactly the same as before. Your circulation will improve, so will your skin and hair, your sense of balance. You will probably sleep better, wake in the mornings feeling completely rested. Your inner organs will work more efficiently; painful periods and chronic indigestion are just two of the problems exercising can help dramatically. Regular exercising will slow down the loss of calcium from bones, so reducing the risk of brittle bones in later years. Because of an increased intake of oxygen you may well find that gradually you are able to think more clearly. And controlled tests have shown that exercise can be a very genuine aid in the treatment of depression.

So exercise can speed you up, sharpen you up and cheer you up. But it can also be very effective at slowing you down. With so many people today leading frenetic lives, learning to slow down now and again is vital if they are not going to get adrenalin burn-out before they reach forty! Tension puts a strain on the heart, raises the blood pressure, causes headaches and allergies – to list but a few of its effects. It can also lead to such disorders as compulsive eating, or under-eating, or to relying on alcohol to make things bearable. Being hyped-up into a 'high' can, under certain circumstances, be not only useful but exhilarating. It can help you face challenges, enable you to deal effectively with certain situations. Your body is ready equipped with the ability to go automatically into a state of red alert for just such emergencies. But the very nature of emergencies is that they are rare. Between times your body needs to wind down, relax, replenish the emotional and physical energy you've used up.

The trouble starts when we spend more time in that state than out of it. After a bit we can become addicted to our stress, looking for problems when things go quiet, anticipating them, even creating them. We have reached a pitch where we need the adrenalin to keep flowing in order to feel alive. Unfortunately, what follows in too many cases is a nervous breakdown, and one of a variety of physical ailments, and in extreme cases, death. And all because we have forgotten how easy and pleasant it is to relax, to completely let go, something that just a little regular exercise would have kept fresh in our minds.

Re-discover your body

Maybe most important of all, though, exercise gets you back in touch with your body. If you're overweight – or think you are! – or very thin, or just unhappy about the way your body is, you've probably taught yourself to ignore it as much as possible. You may even be unaware that you're doing this. Take mirrors. Do you spend the minimum time in front of them, avoid glancing at yourself when you're passing one, even avoid your reflection in windows? Clothes can be another indication. You might find shopping for them a nightmare, do it as rarely as possible, have one favourite outfit such as jeans and bulky sweater, and virtually live in it. On the other hand, you could over-compensate for your dislike of your own body by spending a fortune on clothes, assuming that they will distract attention from what is beneath them.

Many sexual problems stem from a woman being unhappy in her body. Or a man too, for that matter. Often she feels she cannot bear anyone touching her or even close to her. If she's in a relationship, her distrust or dislike of intimacy may result in her withdrawing into herself, rejecting her partner without explaining (or sometimes even understanding) why. A single woman may find herself avoiding making new relationships, lacking confidence in herself, expecting rejection before it happens. Her loneliness may well lead to more disordered eating patterns, more self-disgust. It is only by breaking this spiral that she will be able to see herself for what she is: a unique human being with every right to expect to be loved just exactly as she is. And the first step to breaking the spiral? Getting back in touch with her body. Once she can heighten her sense of body awareness she will begin to regain confidence, even to like herself. Eating the right foods will make her feel better still about it, so will learning how to relax, so will exercising. From then on she'll be a new woman – or the woman she's always been but had forgotten was there.

How much do *you* known about your body, and the way it works?

Our bodies are true miracles, yet we take them for granted. To start with, it's a wonder we manage to stay standing at all. Our two feet cover only a small surface, yet they provide a base on which our bodies are carefully balanced, resisting the force of gravity, not only enabling us to stay upright, but to run, sit, carry heavy weights. What enables our bodies to do this is the fact that though our skeletons are strong and rigid, they are made up of two hundred and six separate bones that allow an amazing variety of movements. These bones are held together by ligaments, but it is the muscles that are responsible for moving them, these receiving their instructions from the nerves, the brain and the spinal cord (through which all messages must pass) which together form the central nervous system for voluntary movements. Good posture allows the body to work efficiently and mostly automatically, the adjustments that need to be made being not only quick and accurate, but also fluid, graceful. When posture is bad both muscles and ligaments will be affected, causing a variety of problems including head and neck aches, misshapen toes, shortage of breath – and, of course, the already mentioned 'middle age spread'. Conversely, good posture can help prevent many of the conditions that are deemed to be automatic as we get older. Arthritis, for example, is an inflammation of the joints caused by a narrowing of the space between the bones in that joint, the most vulnerable being the ones that take the most stress such as hip joints and backbone. A body that moves freely and easily is less likely to have such a problem.

The hormone connection

Because our muscles are also very much involved with the working of our inner organs, keeping them in good condition will also improve a variety of other body functions such as breathing, circulating of blood (the heart itself is a muscle), lymph circulation, digesting food, maintaining body temperature. These are involuntary muscles and are regulated by the sympathetic nervous system, and though their working involves no conscious effort on our behalf, the general condition of our body will undoubtedly have some bearing on how they work. In fact, since the efficiency with which our body functions also has an effect on our hormones which in turn affect our emotions and even our characters, you can see how important it is to keep ourselves fit. Looking good is just an extra plus!

A healthy body, then, is one that works in peak efficiency with the minimum of effort. Which is the way our bodies are designed to work. It is our sedentary way of living coupled with the mental stress that is a fact of life for most people nowadays that causes our bodies to go literally off balance, making us feel permanently tired, giving us difficulty with movement, causing depression and in time, illness.

Sounds gloomy, right? But the good news is that – no matter what your age, how unfit you are, and whether you've spent most of your life doing nothing more energetic than hoovering the house – exercise can work wonders for you, making a change you'll see and feel, and in a comparatively short time, All it takes is a little determination.

Choosing the right exercise

So you don't like exercising. The very thought of it fills you with horror. It brings to mind school hockey matches, all those bruised shins and frozen fingers. Or you tried it once, went to an aerobics class, found yourself angry at the way your body couldn't cope, your face got red. And those changing rooms, packed tight with skinny creatures in orange leotards and purple legwarmers, everyone looking so fit! Or maybe a friend introduced you to tai chi, but it felt rather silly and you got embarrassed. Or you tried jogging and just avoided being hit by a truck. Though most people do take to exercising quite easily once they get started, there are certainly some to whom the prospect is about as appealing as a trip to the dentist. As with the dentist, there is usually some deep-rooted reason for this. If you are such a person, try to think why you feel the way you do. Does it quite simply bore you? Maybe you have so little time to spare you can't see how you could possibly fit it in anyway?

As with changing your attitude to food, the secret is not to try to force yourself to do something you don't want to do, but rather to find the kind of exercise that will give you genuine pleasure. If it doesn't, you'll feel tense and unhappy about it anyway, and many of the benefits will be lost.

Also as with food, your temperament will give you a key to where you might start. With leisure time increasing in the developed countries, there are now many more facilities than ever there were for exercising in a wide variety of ways, some highly concentrated, some so laid back you'll hardly notice you're working, and most of them available to the general public at reasonable prices. There's almost certainly going to be at least one that will suit you. What you have to do is decide which it is, or at least which ones are worth trying.

To help, read carefully through the list below. Under each description of a personality type there are suggestions as to which way of exercising might appeal. Obviously personality types are never this clear cut, and there are other things to be taken into consideration as well – facilities and time available, your age, state of health to start with, not to mention your own personal likes and dislikes! Think of it as a starting point.

You're a loner who is perfectly happy with her own company most of the time, rarely needs other people's approval or encouragement. Once you've made up your mid, you have a fair degree of self-discipline.

If you have the space at home, and a cassette player, you're all set to start your own private exercise class. There are numerous tapes on sale these days, all much of a muchness but the choice is yours. One of the most popular exercises is aerobics, a word that actually refers to anything that is vigorous enough to get you hot and panting (and therefore increases the amount of oxygen you use), but that has come to mean very energetic sessions on the lines of Jane Fonda's original workout. Calisthenics is a less energetic, more stretchy type of routine.

Some tapes combine the two, others add dance exercises, relaxation. A voice will instruct you as to what to do, there is music to help you keep in time (and to make the session less like hard work), and usually a book or chart giving illustrations of each exercise to make sure you get it right. If you've any doubts about a particular exercise, don't do it. It might be worth going to a class for a short while so that you can learn how to do the exercises with an instructor to guide and set you on the right path; doing an exercise incorrectly can be useless – you might even damage yourself.

Yoga is also an ideal system to work on at home. There are countless books to teach you the *asanas* which are a series of postures intended to increase flexibility, reduce tension, improve circulation. Great attention is paid to working on the spine which, in yogic thought, is the key to strength and health. It's best to start with a few simple postures and concentrate on them only, aiming for perfection, before moving onto new ones. Because you take it at your own pace, never forcing your body to do anything it can't, even someone in poor health can benefit from yoga.

An alternative idea for exercising at home is to get one of the many compact exercise machines that are now available at surprisingly reasonable prices. These enable you to cycle a couple of miles per day, to row around a lake, to walk downhill or up a mountain – and all without leaving your living room. Most of them are adjustable so that you can increase the effort you need to make as you gradually become more fit.

You have lots of friends and enjoy being with them as often as possible. In fact, you feel strange if you're not surrounded by people, and need feedback to confirm that you exist at all! In this same category would come someone who – maybe for no fault of their own – has suddenly lost contact with friends and family, who misses the company of others and is feeling lonely.

Social sports are the obvious answer for you. If you want something that isn't too energetic, start with bowls. Golf is another popular sport that will get you out and moving.

Tennis is good for those with more energy to dispose of (or maybe anger – whacking a ball is an excellent therapy when you're furious!). It requires not just a good deal of running about, but a sense of balance, a sharp eye, and good co-ordination. If you've never played before, do have some professional coaching to start with. As with most sports, your playing will benefit, and you'll also be reducing the risk of doing any damage to yourself. Then, for the really energetic, there are squash and badminton, both of which demand that you're in good health before you walk on to the court.

Though all these games can be played in public areas, you will probably find a club you can join not too far from your home. This will mean that you will meet and get to know a set of people with whom you have a least one interest in common. And as all the games are competitive and therefore end with someone winning, there is always the excuse for a celebratory drink at the club bar afterwards.

Maybe you love the outdoors, live in the country or near the sea, or in a city but close to a park that draws you whenever you have free time. The weather doesn't worry you – whatever it's doing it won't stop you, you'll just wrap up in appropriate clothing and get out there.

If a vote was taken on the most popular physical activity of the eighties, it would surely be jogging. Probably its popularity is based on the fact that anyone can do it, it costs next to nothing, there is no special track necessary, you can do it on your own and stop when you like.

An experienced jogger might run four or more miles a day, but even running just a mile can do a great deal of good. Besides being another aerobic exercise (so it's good for your heart, lungs, circulation and stamina) it also helps keep the whole body trim, especially that difficult-to-reach set of muscles of the buttocks. Jogging is also said to actually give you energy. Regular joggers will run even when they arrive home tired, not pushing themselves, allowing the rhythm of their running to gradually calm them, taking in deeper breaths, feeling tension and weariness just fall away. The sense of euphoria some joggers claim to feel is caused by mood-raising chemical reactions in the blood.

Again, do start slowly. For the first week or two run only until you feel any discomfort – shortness of breath, leg cramps – or just tired. Walk until the desire to run again returns. Alternate the walking and running, and in time you'll find it easier and you're going further and faster.

Three important tips to remember. Do a few warm-up stretches and bends both before you start and when you've finished. Wear only proper running shoes – anything else will not give your feet the support they need. Try to find a soft path to run on, preferably away from the dangers of the road, not to mention the fumes!

If jogging doesn't appeal, you could try cycling. This is an excellent form of exercising for the whole body – and has the plus that it gets you from A to B in less time and for free. Because of the ease of movement it is easy to be tempted to over-do it when you first start cycling, something you may only realise when you find yourself a long way from home.

Take care to take it slowly. Comfortable, non-restrictive clothing is essential.

Another possibility for outdoor exercise is horse-riding. This actually is a far more physical activity than one might realise, getting a whole lot of muscles working that you've probably forgotten you've got. Many regular horse-riders, in fact, do some kind of workout as well to keep themselves in shape for their time in the saddle. If you are interested, go along to your local stables and talk to someone about classes. Horse-riding is an expensive way to exercise, but if you've got the money, and the time, and you like horses . . .

You've got lots of energy you need to use up. You work at an office desk, or spend much of your day sitting in a car, or maybe you're just one of those people who are full of bounce. For you, the more energy you use, the more you seem to have. Just the same, the idea of playing some kind of sport doesn't interest you at all, you can't stand clubs, and formal exercise routines remind you too much of school.

How about taking up disco dancing? Though to many youngsters this is considered a pastime and not a form of exercising, it is one of the best ways to strengthen the heart and lungs, to develop balance, to tone legs and arm muscles. In fact, though you won't be concentrating on any specific area, you'll actually be giving your whole body an excellent workout. It's estimated that fifteen minutes of disco dancing is the equivalent to a two mile jog!

Most towns have a least one disco where the music will be energetic and continuous. Don't worry about being watched – you can be sure everyone else will be far too busy doing their own thing to notice what you're doing. You need a partner, of course. Maybe take along your man, or a friend? And wear comfortable shoes or you'll be putting a strain on the wrong parts of your body and could end up limping home.

If you don't like the idea of flinging yourself about in gay abandon in public places, why not find a disco dancing class? This kind of exercise doesn't need to be taught, of course, so any class you attend is unlikely to be very structured or formal.

If you can't find one, how about starting your own with some friends?

As a last resort, there's always your living room. Throw off your inhibitions, put on some music, and dance.

Novelty is the key to capturing your interest. You like the unusual, the exotic, the unexpected. It shows in your home, the clothes you wear, the places you go for your holiday. (Or maybe you don't go away for your holiday, figuring that tourism is ruining the planet!) You're not one of those people who goes out of their way to put across an image of being unconventional – it's just the way you are.

It might well be worth your looking at the martial arts. These Eastern disciplines include aikido, karate, judo and tai chi, and even those come in various styles, some more combative, others slower and more gentle. All are intended to not just strengthen and make the body more flexible, but also to work on the mind. Tai chi in particular – it's sometimes described as meditation in movement. Though not popular with the mass market, they are gradually becoming better known, and there are centres and clubs across the country. Practise them regularly and they may change your whole attitude to life.

If they sound too esoteric for you, how about Spanish dancing? Or belly or Indian dancing? Classes in these might not be easy to find, though they are becoming more widely available too, and will continue to do so as long as there are eccentrics who dare break out of the mould. Though they might sound relatively easy, they are all in fact very intricate, demanding not just a good sense of rhythm but also a healthy body – and if you haven't got one to start with, you will have by the time you've mastered the dance technique. An added dimension is the chance to dress up in appropriate clothing, maybe even to perform in front of an audience.

Gymnastics offer the chance to try some unsual sports. What about javelin or discus throwing, hurdling or the high jump? You may need to find a club at which to learn these skills, and will probably need to do some more basic exercise routine to maintain your fitness level if you have any hopes of reaching a competitive standard.

Or – if you don't mind roughing it, and actually like mud baths – how about taking up rugby? Just as there's no reason why a man shouldn't help out in the kitchen, why shouldn't a woman be allowed to play the team games that up until recently have been reserved for men? All-female rugby, football and cricket teams, though not exactly widespread, are popping up all over the place. If you can't find one locally, why not start your own?

You don't often admit it, but you enjoyed school – the routine, the chance to learn things, being surrounded by familiar faces, having everything you needed under one roof.

A health club would probably suit your temperament well. These can now be found in most localities and – though probably a little more elegant than your school – are similar in that they offer comradeship, tuition and encouragement and a selection of facilities on hand.

A well-equipped club will probably have a gym in which you can use equipment such as the Nautilus (specially designed to work different sets of muscles), bars, weights, and so on. It should also have a swimming pool, maybe a sauna, will hold classes in aerobics, stretch and tone, possibly modern dance. If there is space it will have an outdoor running track which means you can avoid traffic and people walking their dogs; it will also be easier for you to judge how far you have run and therefore note your improvement. There will be professionals on duty at all times to help you use equipment in a way that is safe and most effective. Often such clubs have juice and wholefood bars where you can have a snack of the right kind.

Providing you use it regularly, a health club – though usually quite expensive to join – can be very good value. Most will allow you to look around and have a try out on the equipment before you join. Take advantage of this. Work out how often you would be able to go along, aiming for at least three sessions a week. Then, if you come away with a positive feeling – such places can have the kind of atmosphere that makes you want to start your new regime then and there! – sign on and get down to it. Leisure centres, usually council run, will probably offer a similar selection of facilities, and though the surroundings may be more basic, the fees will be considerably lower.

Self-discipline is not something you're familiar with. You make resolutions and really intend to stick to them, but something happens, or you forget, or are enticed away, and though you always feel rather disappointed in yourself, eventually you give up. You really would like to have more control, and one day you really will make a big effort . . .

You have three alternatives.

One is to give up trying to push yourself into any kind of regular exercise routine, and just do it when the mood takes you. You could vary this – go jogging sometimes, use a tape to do a session at home every now and again, make a point of saying yes if anyone invites you to go swimming or play a game of tennis on the local public courts. You will not get the benefit of exercising regularly, but if you know you're unlikely to be able to stick to such a thing for long, better to at least make an effort to do the little you can.

Or you could join some sort of class – whatever appeals to you – and get someone to join it with you, preferably someone who is very disciplined and who also likes disciplining others.

Failing that, join the most expensive class you can, spend a small fortune on the right clothes and equipment, and hope that you will feel so guilty about the extravagance that you'll feel obliged to go, at least for a time. Then, with a bit of luck, you'll find yourself actually getting fitter – which will be another reason for not giving up.

You're a dare-devil, you love the excitement of doing something that has a degree of risk about it. You see life as a series of challenges and don't feel truly alive unless you're tackling at least one of them at a time, preferably more.

If you carry this philosophy through to all aspects of your life, you are probably a very physical person anyway, and get plenty of exercise – even if it's just rushing about! In fact, it might well be an idea for you to take up yoga, which apart from strengthening your body will also help calm and centre you. Too much excitement can have a similar effect on the body to that of stress in that you could find yourself on a permanent high – which might feel good at the time, but which needs to be balanced with quiet moments.

However, adventure activities are becoming increasingly popular these days. Some are expensive and require specialist equipment – water skiing, for example. Ride the waves for less money by surf-boarding. Hang-gliding is another new fad. Climbing requires skill, a fit body and some equipment; start with some relatively easy climbs and in time if you enjoy it, you'll be able to move on to more difficult gradients with experience to back you – and good strong legs.

Though there are holiday courses available that will give you a taste of many such activities, do try to pick something that you can also continue to enjoy at other times of the year. Spending two weeks climbing in the Welsh mountains can be great fun but it won't do much for your general state of health. Regular exercise is more important than going all out for two weeks, then doing next to nothing for the rest of the year. If there are climbs in your area – even less spectacular ones – make a point of doing them often, and do some exercise routine between times. If you like skiing and have a dry ski run nearby, use it. Don't plan to keep fit by surf-boarding unless you live near a suitable beach.

Time is your problem. There is never enough of it. Everything you do is squeezed in between doing two other things.

Firstly, see the above comments about the value of practising yoga. If your life is really so busy (and not just badly organised) yoga might just save you from having a nervous breakdown. Get up ten minutes earlier, or go to bed ten minutes later – whatever suits you best, as long as you find a tiny space in which to do some regular stretching, relaxing and deep breathing.

In fact, exercising often but for short spaces of time can be as effective as doing longer more concentrated sessions. Some experts think it is *more* effective. Maybe you don't have time to go along to a class or club, or even to do a half hour stretch and tone session in your home. But if you have ten minutes a day to spare – and surely you can find them? – there are plenty of other things you can do instead.

Rebounding is popular in America, and it works. You jump up and down on what is in effect a small trampoline, gradually getting higher, exercising as you bounce, twisting your body, doing jumping jacks and high kicks. Though it sounds simple and need only be as vigorous as you want it to be, this is an aerobic form of exercising. Ten minutes a day will give you a good workout as well as setting the blood racing.

Even simpler, you could try skipping. Keep your rope handy and you can do it whenever you have a few minues to spare – though outdoors is best so that you take in lots of good air. Running shoes are essential if you intend to practise regularly, and make sure you jump and land lightly using the balls of the feet. Skipping also compares well with jogging for its aerobic effect, yet you don't have to find anywhere to run! Less energetic, but very good for the muscles, is isometrics. In brief, this is a system whereby you work the muscles by either pushing and pulling against something, for example, putting the palms of each hand together and then pressing as hard as you can, or simply by contracting them. This means it can be practised anytime, any place. When you're standing in a queue, pull in your stomach and buttocks and hold. When you're waiting for a kettle to boil, reach up and press hard against the top of the door frame. Isometrics won't do much for your heart, breathing or stamina, but it can certainly help tighten muscles so that you look slimmer and feel stronger.

Getting hot and sweaty and tousled is not your idea of having a good time. Or you have some kind of physical disability. Or you're maybe getting on a bit, have never been much of an exerciser or sportswoman, and feel you have a right to take life easy.

Just because you don't want to – or can't – throw yourself into a vigorous programme of exercising doesn't mean you have to give up and opt out. Two of the most perfect exercises of all would be ideal for you.

First, swimming. This is suitable for any age, any state of health. It tones all major muscle groups, has aerobic value when done reasonably briskly, improves circulation, breathing, co-ordination, and because of the weightlessness you experience when the body is supported by water, it's very relaxing. Doctors often actually recommend it as therapy for problems like arthritis and high blood pressure.

You can join a swimming club, but there's no need to. If you have a pool nearby, just make a point of going along regularly – preferably at least a couple of times a week. Start slowly doing two or three laps, resting, doing more laps, and gradually work up to twenty or thirty continuous laps. The crawl is the best stroke for an all-over workout, but most strokes use all muscle groups so just do what you most enjoy.

The other near-perfect exercise is yoga, although not quite perfect because it does not exercise the heart. What it does do is improve suppleness by stretching and compressing muscles, manipulating joints. It also teaches you how to breath properly for maximum energy, works on internal organs such as your stomach, kidneys, and reproductive system, and will relax you. Besides improving your general health, yoga will without doubt affect your whole way of life. It has been practised for many centuries with just that result in mind!

Although there are many excellent books, cassettes and videos available on the subject, yoga is best studied with the aid of a teacher – at least to start with. Make sure you wear loose clothing, have a mat to work on, and that the room is comfortably warm.

Before making up your mind to try any of the above suggestions, do also give careful thought to your own particular lifestyle. Don't try to do the impossible. Preferably choose something that you can do within a short distance of your home, that won't have you too out of pocket before you even get started, and that will still leave you time for friends, your family or budgie, or whatever it is that matters to you most. Certainly it's important to exercise if you want to improve your health, stay in good shape (whatever that shape may be!), look and feel wonderful. But don't let it interfere with other aspects of your life, or become another demand, something else you feel you have to do each day. The intention is for you to enjoy it, not regret ever starting it. If you feel it isn't working, don't see it as a failure, or take it as proof that exercising isn't for you. Instead, just set that idea aside, put it down to experience, and have a go at something else.

Whatever you ultimately choose, do start slowly and carefully. A few simple limbering up stretches and swings before you start can only be beneficial. As your body grows stronger, so you can increase the amount you do. If you haven't exercised for some time, are severly overweight, pregnant or have some problem such as a bad back, do make a point of checking first with your doctor before starting a programme or taking up a sport. Better safe than sorry.

Nothing appeals, not a single one of the above suggestions?

Then try walking more. Just get off the bus a few stops before your destination, or get on it a few stops later. Leave the car at home more often. Make a point of never taking a lift and when you climb the stairs do so briskly. Because walking is something most of us do each day of our lives, we tend to overlook it as a way of keeping fit, yet it is an excellent method, especially if you get away from traffic fumes and can move at a good pace. Besides working on various sets of muscles, improving co-ordination and balance and getting the circulation going, it has the advantage of requiring no equipment, no special time needs to be set aside, and it's free. If you make a habit of walking whenever you can – even just short distances – over a day you will probably find you have covered some miles. Regular exercise of this kind is quite as beneficial as a once-a-week thrash on the squash court – and less likely to cause strains!

It might seem strange, but exercising can also be beneficial for anyone who wants to *put on weight*. Any of the above ideas will give you strength and stamina, help improve both flexibility and posture, keep your heart and circulation working efficiently, all of which will make you feel and look better. Because yoga can be so relaxing, this can slow down your metabolism. As most exceptionally thin people do have very fast metabolic rates, this will undoubtedly help. Weightlifting is another good idea for the underweight. Not only can it fill out the muscles, making you appear to be more full-bodied, but large muscles weigh more.

Though this chapter may appear to have been specifically written for women, that does not mean the man in your life will not also benefit enormously from committing himself to some kind of regular exercise programme. Most of the suggestions would apply equally well to a man, though he might be more drawn to working in a gymnasium, or with weights, or to playing tennis rather than taking up belly dancing!

If you're about to start something new, and it's appropriate, why not get him to join you? The big new changes you're about to make in your lifestyle will very much affect your whole life – how much better if you can share the experience with someone close to you.

Note: Remember, anyone who has not exercised for some time, is severely overweight, suffers from any illness, is taking medicine, or is just unsure, would be well advised to see a doctor or practitioner in alternative medicine before starting regular exercising. *Everyone* should remember to start slowly, doing only as much as is comfortable. In time your body will become fitter and you will be able to do more without risking straining, or doing more serious damage.

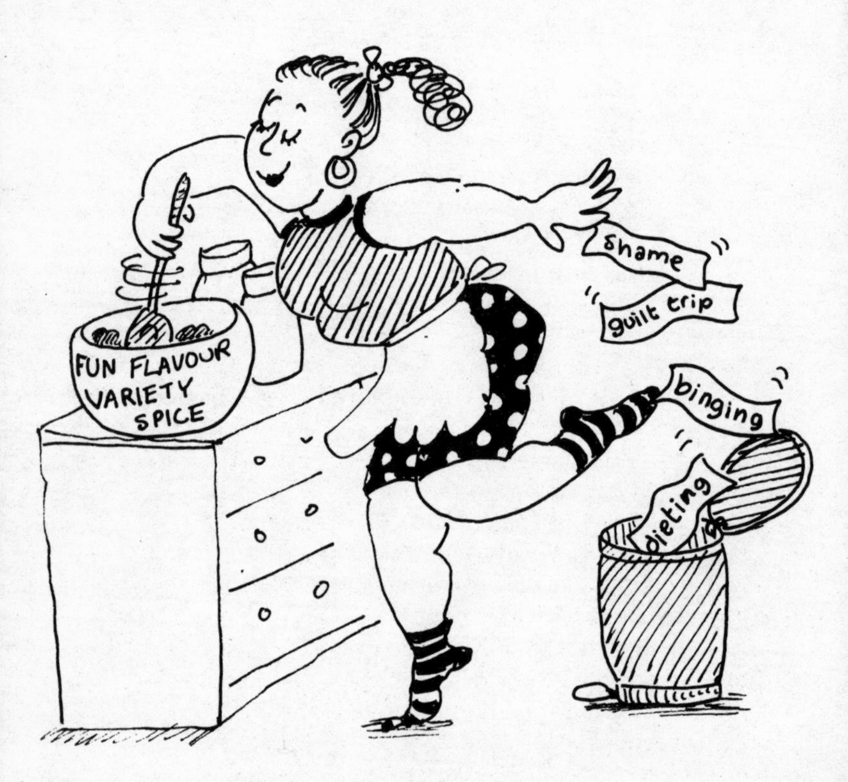

Food will become a pleasure again

8 *R*ecipes for success

So you're getting the idea.

You've thought a lot about the way you eat and have resolved to give up the guilt trip, to put aside fear, and – if necessary – to do something about those habits and attitudes you've been lugging about since childhood. Your intention is to learn to enjoy again the simple foods that taste good and do you good – or at least, the minimum harm. You've signed a peace treaty with your body. No more brow-beating it into submission, no more anger. No more being ashamed of the way you look, either; you wouldn't let anyone tell you what curtains to put up, what colour to paint your kitchen, so why let them dictate how you should look? No matter whether you're voluptuous or all bones, if *you're* happy with your body, that's all that matters. And when you eat healthily, find time to relax, and take regular exercise in whatever way gives you most pleasure, you *will* be!

Best of all, you'll be free once and for all from the need to be forever worrying about what you should and shouldn't eat. You'll no longer be obsessed. Think of it – food will become a pleasure again.

Using wholefoods isn't nearly as complicated as is rumoured, but you may need to adjust some of your ideas. Forget about a balanced meal being a slab of meat and two over-cooked veg. Look instead at other cuisines where a variety of ingredients are combined in unusual and imaginative ways, yet the resulting meals provide a good balance of nutrients. Use such cuisines as a starting point for devising meals of your own, keeping in mind tastes and textures as well as nourishment. Balance a hot pasta dish with a crisp and crunchy salad. Follow a bean soup with a soufflé, or vegetables in a light sauce. If you want to serve a specially rich dessert, maybe start your meal with a dish based on tofu and beansprouts. Or looking at it the other way round, don't serve a spiced soup before a curry, nor a chilled one before a salad (not in winter, anyway), nor a creamed vegetable one before a vegetables in cream sauce dish. Sounds obvious, but it's amazing how many people forget about balance. Heavy and light, hot and cold, sweet and sour, smooth and crisp – ring the changes.

We all eat with our eyes, too. Looking at what we're about to eat is a very pleasant prelude; it gives us a moment in which to tingle with anticipation, and for the saliva to start flowing. Colour is important here. Again, try for variety, making a point of adding something to liven up the look of a dish. This is where garnishes come in useful. They may seem fiddly, but they need not be. A few slices of tomato or cucumber, chopped celery leaves, some golden croûtons, flaked and roasted nuts, and herbs of all kinds can be used to top a dish just before serving.

To get you started

On the following pages you'll find suggested meal plans for four separate weeks, one for each season of the year. Below them are recipes for each of the items marked with an asterisk. Included are ideas for special occasions such as a dinner party, a buffet party, a picnic, and Christmas lunch – just to show that eating healthily doesn't have to mean no more celebratory meals.

Unlike the suggestions you'll find in other books on dieting, these do not have to be followed religiously. The aim is simply to show you how basic ingredients can be used and combined to make delicious meals. Use the plans in whatever way suits you best. Dip into them as and when you want, taking a recipe from one, serving it with a dish from another day or even another week. Use vegetable and salad ingredients often, varying them as much as your local shops allow. Nowadays, what with extended growing seasons, items being imported from around the world, and the variety of good quality frozen vegetables that can be found in most shops, it is possible to have courgettes mid-winter, leeks in summer! Though quantities should be sufficient for four, do adjust them to suit yourself, your family – and everyone's appetites. These vary enormously, one person's snack seeming like a gargantuan feast to another. Only by using the recipes will you be able to tell. Most wholefood dishes will keep for a day or two in the fridge, so if you make too much, use the extra to make a soup or stew another day.

Treat the plans also as a framework on which you can base your own balanced eating plans, using the ingredients and dishes you like best. Just remember the three-way path.

1. Use good, wholesome foods.
2. Vary them.
3. Relax and enjoy!

Spring

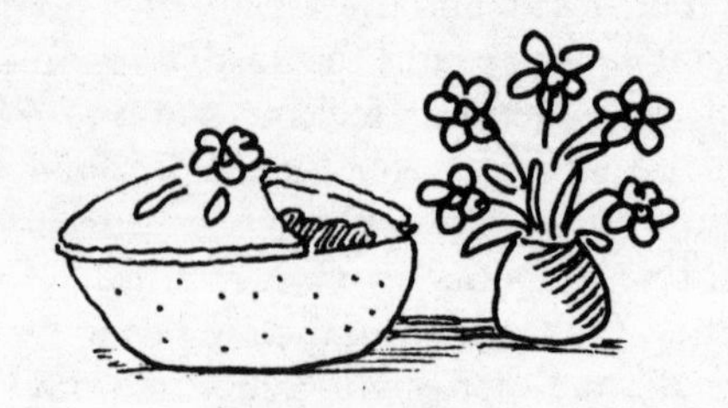

BREAKFAST	LUNCH	DINNER
Day 1		
Fresh or frozen orange juice Wheatflakes with soya or dairy milk Herb tea or decaffeinated coffee	Broccoli and hazelnut soup* Wholemeal roll Tomato and watercress salad	Macaroni and vegetable bake in tahini or cheese sauce Raw cauliflower salad Fresh fruit salad
Day 2		
Apple juice Maple apricot granola* with soya or dairy milk Herb tea or decaffeinated coffee	Mixed salad with aduki beans Hot muffins Carton of plain yogurt	Spring vegetable pie* New potatoes Lightly steamed spinach Rhubarb crumble
Day 3		
Half a grapefruit Wholemeal toast with marmalade or honey Herb tea or decaffeinated coffee	Walnut and pepper pâté* French bread Pasta salad Fresh fruit	Pancakes filled with celery and walnuts in white or tomato sauce Green salad Tahini biscuits*

Day 4

Mixed fruit juice
Muesli with soya or dairy milk
Herb tea or decaffeinated coffee

Three bean salad
Raw spinach and mushroom salad
Corn bread*

Cashew stir-fried rice*
Courgettes in yogurt
Watercress
Fresh fruit salad

Day 5

Grapefruit juice
Wholemeal bread with real fruit jam or honey
Herb tea or decaffeinated coffee

Deep-fried mushrooms with avocado sauce*
Mixed green salad
Rye crackers
Wholemeal hot cross buns

Beansprout omelette
Spring cabbage
Steamed new potatoes
Fresh fruit

Day 6

Fruit juice and tofu shake
Wholemeal toast with tahini
Herb tea or decaffeinated coffee

Minestrone with semolina dumplings and/or grated cheese
Tomato salad
Dried fruit bar

Chili kidney beans
Bulgar or other grain
Baked apples with cream or concentrated soya milk

Day 7

Orange juice
Oatcakes with yeast extract, honey or cheese
Herb tea or decaffeinated coffee

Nutburger on wholemeal bap
Chutney, coleslaw
Carton of plain yogurt

Special occasion dinner (vegan)
Cream of asparagus soup*
Chinese leaves with tofu*
Sesame noodles*
Watercress salad*
Fruit tartlets with coconut cream*

BROCCOLI AND HAZELNUT SOUP

1 tablespoon vegetable oil
1 small onion, peeled and sliced
455g (1 lb) broccoli, washed and broken into florets
55g (2oz) hazelnuts, ground
1 tablespoon chopped lemon peel
1.15 litres (2 pints) vegetable stock
seasoning to taste
½–1 teaspoon curry powder
plain yogurt, concentrated soya milk or single cream – optional
2 tablespoons coarsely chopped hazelnuts (preferably roasted)*

Heat the oil and gently fry the onion for a few minutes. Put into a liquidiser with the broccoli, ground nuts, lemon peel, curry powder and seasoning and blend to make a thick purée. Add more stock as necessary.

Transfer to a saucepan and heat very gently, stirring occasionally. Check the seasoning and adjust if necessary. Pour into four bowls, add a swirl of yogurt, soya milk or cream if liked. Sprinkle with the chopped nuts.

*To dry-roast any nuts put them in a pan and cook over a medium heat, moving them about to stop burning, until they begin to colour and smell cooked. When cool enough, rub off the skins and use as necessary. They can also be oven roasted.

MAPLE APRICOT GRANOLA

6 tablespoons vegetable oil
6 tablespoons maple syrup
680g (1½ lbs) mixed cereal flakes
115g (4oz) sunflower seeds
115g (4oz) almonds, coarsely chopped
115g (4oz) flaked coconut
the peel of 1 orange, coarsely sliced
55g (2oz) sesame seeds
225g (8oz) dried apricot pieces

In a pan, and over a gentle heat, mix the oil and syrup. Then stir in the cereal flakes, making sure they are evenly coated. Add the sunflower seeds, almonds and flaked coconut.

Spread the mixture in one or two large baking tins. Cook at

300°F/150°C (Gas Mark 2) for 30 minutes, stirring now and again. Mix in the orange peel and sesame seeds, cook approximately 10 minutes more. The granola is cooked when it begins to colour and goes crisp. Remove from the heat, stir in the chopped apricot pieces, and leave to cool.

Store the granola in a large screw-top jar and use as needed, either as a breakfast cereal, or as a topping for fruit salad or ice cream.

SPRING VEGETABLE PIE

Pastry:
225g (8oz) wholemeal flour
good pinch of salt
115g (4oz) chilled butter or vegetarian 'lard'
1 dessertspoon lemon juice
approx. 4 tablespoons ice-cold water

Filling:
1 small cauliflower, broken into florets
2 tablespoons vegetable oil
1 small bunch spring onions, cut into chunks
2 small courgettes, sliced
115g (4oz) mushrooms, sliced
1 tablespoon wholemeal flour
200ml (1/3 pint) single cream or concentrated soya milk
seasoning to taste
approx. 4 tablespoons cooked kidney beans – optional

Sift together the flour and salt, then use a knife to cut the fat into very small pieces and stir into the flour. Mix lemon juice and water and add to the flour and fat, working quickly with cool hands. Wrap the lumpy dough in a polythene bag and leave in the fridge for 30 minutes.

Meanwhile, prepare the filling. Steam the cauliflower for a few minutes. In a separate pan, heat the oil and gently fry the onions, courgettes and mushrooms, turning them every now and again. Add the drained cauliflower.

Sprinkle the flour onto the vegetables, cook briefly, stir in the cream or soya milk and continue cooking until the sauce thickens. Season to taste. If you have some kidney beans handy (or any other kind!) stir these into the vegetables. Pile into an overproof dish.

On a floured board, and again working quickly, roll out the pastry as thinly as possible. Lay it across the vegetables, trim, and press down the edges. Prick the top with a fork.

Bake at 400°F/200°C (Gas Mark 6) for about 15 minutes or until cooked.

WALNUT AND PEPPER PÂTÉ

115g (4oz) low-fat cream cheese
4 tablespoons plain yogurt
½ small red pepper, finely chopped
½ small green pepper, finely chopped
55g (2oz) walnut pieces, coarsely ground or finely chopped
seasoning to taste
1 tablespoon chopped chives
good pinch of paprika
extra paprika and watercress to decorate

Blend together the cheese and yogurt, then gradually add all the other ingredients. The mixture should be heavy to stir – if it's too runny add more cheese or nuts.

Press the mixture into a small dish, smooth the top, and chill for at least 30 minutes before using. A little extra paprika and a sprig or two of watercress add colour to the pâté.

TAHINI BISCUITS

2 tablespoons tahini (sesame paste)
55g (2oz) margarine
55g (2oz) raw cane suger
1 free-range egg
115g (4oz) wholemeal flour
2 teaspoons baking powder
1 teaspoon mixed spice, or to taste
55g (2oz) currants
1–2 tablespoons sesame seeds – optional

Cream together the tahini, margarine and sugar until thoroughly blended. Lightly whisk the egg and add.

Sift together the flour, baking powder and spice, and stir this into the mixture. Add the currants. Using floured hands, divide the dough into 12 small, even-sized balls. Arrange them on an ungreased baking tray leaving space for them to spread, and press down gently with the back of a spoon. Sprinkle each one lightly with some sesame seeds, press down again.

Bake at 350°F/180°C (Gas Mark 4) for 15 to 20 minutes, or until crisp and golden. Allow to cool slightly, then transfer to a wire rack and leave until completely cold.

CORN BREAD

115g (4oz) maize (corn) flour
115g (4oz) wholemeal flour
3 teaspoons baking powder
good pinch of salt
1 tablespoon vegetable oil
2 flat tablespoons honey
1 free-range egg – optional
approx. 200ml (1/3 pint) water, milk or buttermilk

Sift the two flours, baking powder and salt together in a bowl.

Combine the oil and honey over a low heat, stir well, add to the dry ingredients. If using, stir in the lightly whisked egg.

Add just enough liquid to make a soft, thick batter. Stir well, then pour into a small greased cake tin and bake at 350°F/180°C (Gas Mark 4) for about 30 minutes. To test if the corn bread is done, press fingers lightly in the centre – it should feel firm.

Leave to cool, cut into squares and serve.

CASHEW STIR-FRIED RICE

3 tablespoons vegetable oil
1/2 clove of garlic, crushed
1 medium onion, chopped
2 sticks of celery, chopped
115g (4oz) mushrooms, sliced
115g (4oz) mange tout, trimmed
115g (4oz) baby sweetcorn, washed
85g (3oz) cashew nuts
soy sauce
good squeeze of lemon juice
2 cups cooked brown rice

watercress

Heat 2 tablespoons of the oil and gently fry the garlic, onion and celery until they begin to soften. Add another spoonful of oil and stir in the remaining vegetables and nuts. Continue cooking, stirring continually, for another 5 minutes or so. Sprinkle generously with soy sauce and lemon juice.

The rice should be well drained before using. This is an excellent way to use up left-overs! Stir it into the pan and contnue cooking gently until it is hot. You may need to add more oil or soy sauce if the mixture gets too dry.

Serve at once with watercress garnish.

DEEP-FRIED MUSHROOMS WITH AVOCADO SAUCE

Sauce:
1 large ripe avocado, stoned and peeled
140ml (1/4 pint) plain yogurt
1 tablespoon chopped parsley
1 tablespoon chopped chives
garlic salt to taste
small piece of raw onion – optional
1 tablespoon lemon juice
seasoning to taste
Mushrooms:
85g (3oz) wholemeal flour
good pinch of salt
1 1/2 tablespoons vegetable oil
7 tablespoons warm water
the white of 1 free-range egg
170g (6oz) button mushrooms, washed and dried
extra flour
vegetable oil for deep frying

As the sauce needs to be chilled, it is best made in advance. Either mash the avocado and mix in all the other ingredients, making the sauce as smooth as possible, or use a blender. Leave covered until needed. Adjust the taste and texture if necessary.

Sift together the flour and salt, add the oil and warm water. Whisk the egg white until very stiff and then fold this into the mixture. Dust the mushrooms with flour, dip them into the batter mix, and deep-fry a small batch in hot oil until golden. Drain well and keep them warm whilst cooking the remaining mushrooms.

CREAM OF ASPARAGUS SOUP

2 tablespoons vegetable oil
1 small onion, finely chopped
340g (12oz) fresh asparagus, finely chopped*
850ml (1½ pints) vegetable stock
good pinch of nutmeg
1 teaspoon parsley
good pinch dry dill
good pinch dry tarragon
seasoning to taste
4 tablespoons concentrated soya milk or tahini

Heat the oil and gently fry the onion and asparagus for a few minutes. Cover with stock, add the nutmeg, and cook until the vegetables are soft.

Blend well, add herbs and seasoning. Bring gently back to the boil and divide between four small bowls. Stir a spoonful of soya milk or tahini in each one just before serving.

*Asparagus is very expensive – unless you have your own private source. If not, look out for the thin stems called 'sprew' that are often cheaper than the larger ones and are perfect for use in soups.

CHINESE LEAVES WITH TOFU

3 tablespoons vegetable oil
285g (10oz) tofu, cubed*
4 tablespoons ginger wine, or to taste
1 tablespoon soy sauce
1 teaspoon raw cane suger
285ml (½ pint) vegetable stock
1 good tablespoon cornflour
1 large red pepper, sliced
1 medium head Chinese leaves, coarsely shredded
115g (4oz) mung bean sprouts
seasoning to taste
parsley

Heat the oil and gently fry the tofu cubes, turning them so that all sides are slightly coloured. Mix together the ginger wine, soy sauce and sugar, and add to the pan with most of the stock. Bring to a slow boil.

Stir the cornflour into the remaining stock and add, continuing to cook until the sauce begins to thicken. Add the pepper and Chinese leaves, stir well. Cook briefly until the vegetables begin to soften, then add the bean sprouts and cook for just a few minutes more. Season to taste, serve hot with parsley garnish.

*Tofu should be removed from the pack, rinsed in cold water, then wrapped in something like a clean tea towel and left for at least half an hour with a weight on top. This extracts all the moisture, giving the tofu a firmer texture. Silken tofu is a softer tofu altogether, and better used in dips and sweets.

SESAME NOODLES

285g (10oz) Chinese noodles
1 tablespoon vegetable oil, preferably sesame
small piece of fresh root ginger, peeled and finely chopped
30g (1oz) sesame seeds
black pepper

The noodles will need to be cooked in boiling water for a short time – check instructions on pack. When just tender, drain them well and set aside.

Heat the oil and add the ginger, cook briefly. Add the seeds and cook a little longer. Stir in the noodles and continue cooking gently until heated through. Good with freshly ground black pepper.

WATERCRESS SALAD

1 bunch watercress, washed and broken into sprigs
1 cucumber, peeled and thinly sliced
4 medium tomatoes, quartered
55g (2oz) walnut pieces
1 small endive or crisp lettuce
Dressing:
1 tablespoon tarragon or wine vinegar
3 tablespoons vegetable oil, preferably walnut

1 teaspoon English mustard
seasoning to taste

Mix the watercress, cucumber, tomatoes and walnuts together. Combine the ingredients for the salad dressing (easiest to do by putting them into a small screw-top bottle and shaking well!). Pour some over the mixed ingredients, toss gently.

Arrange the salad in the centre of a bed of endive or lettuce. Put extra salad dressing on the table for anyone who wants more.

FRUIT TARTLETS WITH COCONUT CREAM

Pastry:
170g (6oz) wholemeal flour
85g (3oz) margarine
good squeeze of lemon juice
2–3 tablespoons cold water
Filling:
small strawberries
grapes
kiwi fruits
200ml (1/3 pint) water
1 teaspoon rosewater
1 teaspoon raw cane sugar
Cream:
115g (4oz) block creamed coconut
boiling water
vanilla essence or rosewater – optional

To make the pastry, put the flour into a bowl and use fingertips to rub in the fat to make a crumb-like mixture. Mix lemon juice and water and add to the flour, kneading briefly to make a firm dough. Wrap this in a polythene bag, put into the fridge, chill for 30 minutes.

Roll out the dough and cut into eight circles, using these to line small tins. Press the pastry down firmly, prick the bases. Bake blind at 400°F/200°C (Gas Mark 6) for 10 minutes then set aside to cool.

Wash the fruit, dry well. Fill each tartlet with strawberries and grapes, decorate the tops with slices of kiwi fruit. In a small saucepan gently heat the water, rosewater and sugar, stirring often, and continue simmering until the sauce thickens and clears.

Cool slightly, then pour some over the top of each of the tarts, spreading it so that all the fruit is covered. Leave to get cold.

Grate the coconut and add just enough boiling water to make a thick cream. Flavour with vanilla or rosewater, if liked. Leave the cream to get cold then top each tartlet with a spoonful or two. If you prefer to put it on the table for people to help themselves, add a drop of hot water and stir again just before serving – when cold it tends to firm up.

Summer

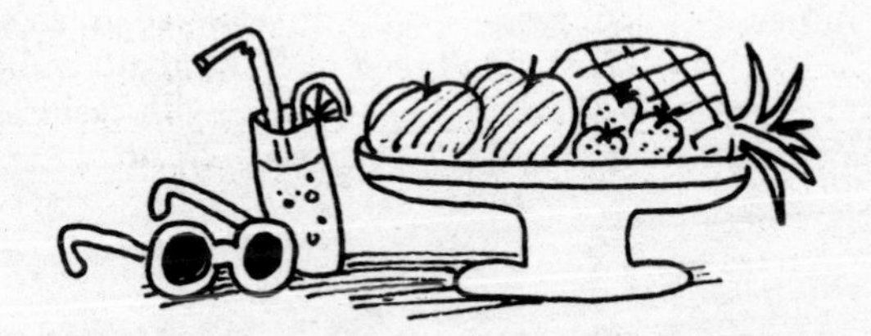

BREAKFAST	LUNCH	DINNER
Day 1		
Dried fruit compôte with natural yogurt Crispbread Herb tea or decaffeinated coffee	Carrot soup Mixed salad with tinned nutmeat Wholemeal roll	Stuffed peppers* Jacket potatoes Steamed green beans Fresh fruit
Day 2		
Orange juice Bran muffins with honey or low sugar jam Herb tea or decaffeinated coffee	Green salad with nuts, raisins, banana chunks Tofu dressing* French bread	Cauliflower cheese soufflé New potatoes Ratatouille Stewed mixed fruits
Day 3		
½ melon Wholemeal baps with yeast extract Herb tea or decaffeinated coffee	Pasta salad with fennel, carrot, cucumber and peas Small carton plain yogurt	Shepherds pie Spinach Tomato salad Fruit fool made with egg whites

Day 4

Summer fruit muesli* Bread and nut butter Herb tea or decaffeinated coffee	Mint hummus* Raw vegetable fingers Warm pita bread	Aubergine and ricotta lasagne* Mixed green salad Rhubarb crumble with cashew cream

Day 5

Apricot and lemon juice Scrambled eggs on toast Herb tea or decaffeinated coffee	Chilled lettuce soup Bean pâté and cucumber sandwiches Dried fruit bar	Spiced cauliflower* Courgette and red pepper salad Hot grain dish such as wheat berries Fresh fruit salad

Day 6

Apple juice Oat flakes with soya or dairy milk Herb tea or decaffeinated coffee	Breaded tofu cutlets (fried) Celery sticks Wholemeal baps	Pizza with mushrooms, pepper, olives, sunflower seeds and cheese Green salad Fresh raspberry sorbet*

Day 7

Orange and grapefruit segments Toasted bran raisin muffins Herb tea or decaffeinated coffee	*Summer picnic* Sunflower croquettes* Wholemeal baps* Raw vegetable fingers Flageolet dip* Tortilla chips and crisps Potato and broad bean salad Sesame carob squares* Carrot muffins* Dried fruit and nut mix Fresh fruit	Aubergine and chick pea casserole Green salad Fresh fruit salad

STUFFED PEPPERS

2 large green peppers
2 large red peppers
2 tablespoons vegetable oil
1 medium onion, sliced
1 clove of garlic, crushed
1 large courgette, coarsely chopped
2 large tomatoes, coarsely chopped
140ml (1/4 pint) vegetable stock
4 tablespoons soy bean flakes, soaked in hot water*
approx. 1/2 teaspoon dried mixed herbs
seasoning to taste
85g (3oz) cheddar cheese, grated (optional)
2 tablespoons wholemeal breadcrumbs

Cut the top off the peppers, remove the seeds, and steam them for about 10 minutes until just tender. Turn them upside down and leave standing on a rack to drain well.

Heat the oil and gently fry the onion and garlic to soften. Add the courgette and tomatoes with the stock and bring to the boil. Sprinkle in the drained soy bean flakes, stir well, simmer the mixture for 10 minutes. The liquid should have been soaked up, but if not, drain off any excess. Add herbs and seasoning to taste.

Stand the peppers side by side in a small overproof dish and stuff them with the soy bean and vegetable mix. Sprinkle some grated cheese over the top of each one if liked.

Bake at 375°F/190°C (Gas Mark 5) for 20 minutes. Top the peppers with breadcrumbs and put them under the grill until the crumbs are brown and crisp.

*Soy bean flakes not only give this stuffing mix an unusual texture, but make it high in protein. If you cannot get them, use lentils or bulgar instead.

TOFU DRESSING

225g (8oz) tofu, rinsed and pressed
2 tablespoons oil, preferably olive
1 tablespoon tahini
1 tablespoon lemon juice
1–2 teaspoons honey
seasoning to taste

Use a liquidiser to combine all the ingredients. The dressing should be creamy and smooth. Adjust the consistency, if necessary, and check the seasoning.

SUMMER FRUIT MUESLI (for one)

1 tablespoon rolled oats, soaked overnight in water
1 teaspoon lemon juice
1 tablespoon hazelnuts or almonds, coarsely ground
1 tablespoon raw cane sugar or honey – optional
3 tablespoons plain yogurt
3 tablespoons fresh fruit (i.e. raspberries, cherries, strawberries, sliced apricots – or a mixture)

Simply combine all the ingredients, adding a generous amount of fruit to the muesli just before you are ready to eat.

The original muesli was a fruit dish with just a small amount of grain added. You can use this as a basic recipe and adapt it to include other fruits – apples, pears, bananas, for example. Try it also with different grains, and with soya or dairy milk instead of yogurt.

MINT HUMMUS

455g (1 lb) chick peas, soaked overnight (or use tinned)
3 tablespoons lemon juice
1 clove of garlic, peeled and crushed
good pinch of cumin
3 tablespoons tahini
1–2 tablespoons olive oil
1–2 tablespoons chopped fresh mint
seasoning to taste

mint sprigs to garnish

Pour away the liquid in which the chick peas were soaked. Put them into a pan with fresh water, bring to a fast boil and continue boiling for 10 minutes. Then lower the heat, cover the pan, and cook until tender. This can take 45 minutes to an hour. Cool, then drain, reserving the water.

Use a grinder to powder the chick peas. Or you can do this by hand with a mortar and pestle, or fork, but be prepared to work hard – also for the hummus to be less smooth.

Mix in the other ingredients, taste and adjust as necessary. The hummus should be the consistency of a thick cream. If necessary, add a drop of the liquid in which the chick peas were cooked. Pile into a small dish, smooth the top, garnish with mint sprigs.

Any uneaten hummus will keep for a few days in the fridge.

AUBERGINE AND RICOTTA LASAGNE

1 large aubergine, cut into thin slices
170g (6oz) lasagne
3 tablespoons vegetable oil
1 onion, sliced
6 tomatoes, peeled and chopped (or tinned equivalent)
½–1 teaspoon dried oregano
2 tablespoons tomato purée
seasoning to taste
225g (8oz) ricotta cheese, crumbled
115g (4oz) mozzarella cheese, sliced

Lay the aubergine slices on a plate and sprinkle with salt. After 30 minutes, rinse them with fresh water and pat dry. This will remove the bitter taste.

Bring a large pan of water to the boil, add a tablespoonful of oil, then drop the lasagne sheets in one by one and cook for the time indicated on the pack. Remove them from the pan, rinse with cold water, then lay them flat on a clean tea towel. You can now also buy lasagne that doesn't need to be cooked first, in which case ignore this step.

Use 2 tablespoons of oil and fry the aubergine slices, turning them when one side is cooked. Set aside to drain.

In the remaining oil, cook the onion until soft. Add the tomatoes, oregano, tomato purée and seasoning, and cook gently to make a thick but moist sauce. If necessary, add water or vegetable stock.

Grease a shallow tin or overproof dish. Spread just a little of the tomato sauce across the base and cover with a third of the lasagne sheets. Spread half the ricotta over this, half the aubergine slices, more tomato sauce and then another layer of lasagne. Repeat this. Finish with some more tomato sauce and then the mozzarella cheese slices. When using lasagne that has not been pre-cooked, you need to make sure the lasagne sheets are well covered with sauce – make up some extra if necessary.

Cover with foil or a lid. Bake at 375°F/190°C (Gas Mark 5) for about 30 minutes. Take off the lid and cook for a further 5 minutes.

SPICED CAULIFLOWER

2 tablespoons vegetable oil
½ teaspoon ground coriander
½ teaspoon ground cumin
½ teaspoon ground turmeric
pinch cayenne pepper
1 good tablespoon wholemeal flour
1 onion, sliced
2 medium cauliflowers, broken into large florets
1 large carrot, diced
1 large cooking apple, diced
cold water
seasoning to taste
140g (5oz) carton sour cream or plain yogurt
4 hard-boiled free-range eggs or 4 tablespoons cooked chick peas
fresh parsley

Heat the oil and gently cook the spices for just a few minutes, stirring frequently. Add the flour and cook a minute more. Stir in the onion, cauliflower, carrot and apple, plus just enough water to cover. Bring to the boil, cover the pan and cook gently for about 10 minutes, or until the vegetables are just cooked.

Season to taste, add the sour cream or yogurt, return the pan to a low heat for a few minutes more. Either stir in the quartered eggs or the chick peas, or transfer the cauliflower to a serving dish and put the eggs or peas on top. Add lots of parsley for colour.

FRESH RASPBERRY SORBET

340g (12oz) fresh raspberries
170g (6oz) raw cane sugar
200ml (1/3 pint) water
the whites of 2 free-range eggs

Put the raspberries into a pan with the sugar and water and cook gently, stirring often, until the sugar dissolves. Leave to cool, then rub through a sieve to make a purée. Pour into a freezing tray and freeze until just becoming slushy, then turn out and fold into the stiffly beaten egg whites.

Freeze for a few hours. Remove from the freezer 5 to 10 minutes before needed so that the sorbet softens, but take care it doesn't melt - probably best left in the fridge, especially on a hot day.

If you prefer, you can add the egg whites before freezing, but the above method gives the sorbet a lighter texture.

SUNFLOWER CROQUETTES

115g (4oz) sunflower seeds, ground
115g (4oz) fine wholemeal breadcrumbs
3 spring onions, finely chopped
1 stick of celery, finely chopped
1 carrot, coarsely grated
approx. 140ml (1/4 pint) vegetable stock
1 tablespoon tahini
wheatgerm, bran, sesame seeds or crushed Weetabix to coat

Mix together all the ingredients, making sure they are thoroughly blended. The mixture should be thick but not too dry so adjust the texture, if necessary, by adding more stock or tahini. Divide into equal-sized portions and shape into croquettes. Roll each one in your choice of coating ingredient.

Arrange the croquettes on a baking sheet and bake at 350°F/180°C (Gas Mark 4) for 15 to 20 minutes, turning them occasionally. Leave to cool.

WHOLEMEAL BAPS

455g (1 lb) wholemeal flour
good pinch of salt
just under 30g (1oz) fresh yeast (or ½ oz dried yeast)
1 teaspoon vegetable oil
just under 285ml (½ pint) warm water

Mix the flour and salt. Cream the yeast with a little water and set aside until it begins to froth. Add it to the flour together with the oil and most of the water, mixing well. As you knead the dough check the consistency and add the rest of the water if necessary (the dough should be thick and elastic). Return it to the warmed bowl, cover with a tea towel and leave in a warm place until doubled in size.

With floured hands break into 4 to 6 even-sized pieces, roll into balls and then flatten these slightly. Arrange on a greased baking tray, dust with more flour. Cover lightly and leave in the warmth for about 10 minutes or until nicely risen.

Bake at 400°F/200°C (Gas Mark 6) for 15 to 20 minutes. Transfer to a wire rack and leave to cool. Put a cloth over them to help the insides stay soft.

FLAGEOLET DIP

225g (8oz) flageolets, soaked overnight
115g (4oz) dairy or tofu mayonnaise
squeeze of lemon juice
seasoning to taste
fresh mint and chives

Drain off the soaking water and put the flageolets in a pan with fresh water. Bring to the boil, boil for 10 minutes, then lower the heat, cover, and simmer for about 45 minutes, or until soft. Drain well.

Use a blender to purée the beans, or mash them with a fork. Gradually stir in the other ingredients, adjust taste as necessary. Chill briefly.

Flageolets are expensive because they are picked when young – in fact, their delicate taste is more like fresh beans than that of any of the other dried varieties, which is what makes them special. Use a good quality mayonnaise in this dip so as not to swamp that taste – or mix the mayonnaise with quark, sour cream or yogurt to dilute it, or use any of these instead of mayonnaise.

SESAME CAROB SQUARES

140g (5oz) sesame seeds
55g (2oz) desiccated coconut
2 tablespoons peanut butter
2 tablespoons raw cane sugar
2 tablespoons honey or maple syrup
½ teaspoon vanilla essence
2 tablespoons carob powder

Combine all the ingredients, mixing well. Press into a well greased tin – the mixture should be about ½″ in thickness.

Bake at 300°F/150°C (Gas Mark 2) for 10 to 15 minutes. Mark into squares but leave to cool for a while before cutting. Best made the day before you need them so that they have time to set firm.

CARROT MUFFINS

2 free-range eggs, well beaten
55g (2oz) raw cane sugar
140ml (¼ pint) vegetable oil
1 large cooking apple, peeled and grated
2 medium carrots, peeled and grated
55g (2oz) sultanas
55g (2oz) walnut pieces
170g (6oz) wholemeal flour
2 teaspoons baking powder
½ teaspoon ground cinnamon
½ teaspoon mixed spice

Add the eggs to the sugar and oil and beat until smooth. Stir in the carrot, apple, sultanas and walnuts.

Sift the dry ingredients together and use a metal spoon to fold these lightly into the first mixture.

Grease 12 muffin tins. Fill each tin two-thirds full. Bake at 375°F/190°C (Gas Mark 5) for 15 minutes, or until well risen and golden.

Autumn

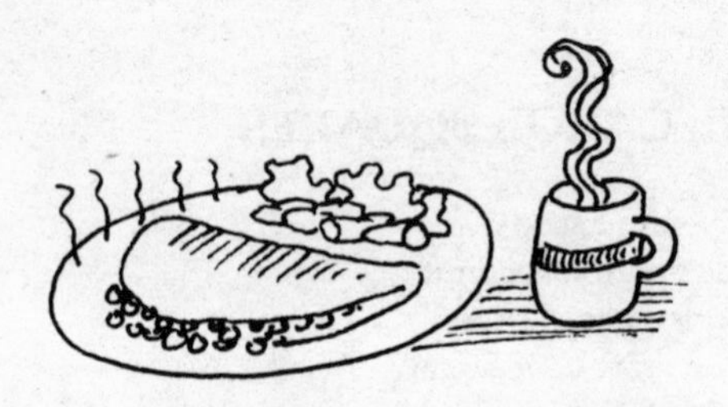

BREAKFAST	LUNCH	DINNER
Day 1		
Grapefruit juice Bran flakes with sultanas and soya or diary milk Herb tea or decaffeinated coffee	Borscht (beetroot soup)* Rye bread Mixed salad with slices of hard-boiled egg	Leek and almond crumble* Jacket potatoes Watercress Hot apple purée
Day 2		
Pineapple juice Toast with tahini Herb tea or decaffeinated coffee	Salad with beansprouts, Chinese leaves, pineapple chunks and roasted peanuts Bran muffin	Spanish quiche* Carrots with parsley Roast potatoes Fresh fruit
Day 3		
One orange Three-seed muesli with soya or dairy milk Herb tea or decaffeinated coffee	Wholemeal sandwiches with peanut butter, low fat cream cheese and celery One banana	Creamed sweetcorn pancakes* Mixed green salad Rice salad Melon and grape dessert

Day 4

Mixed fruit juice
Shredded wheat with soya or dairy milk
Herb tea or decaffeinated coffee

Marrow ratatouille with smoked tofu*
Fresh fruit

Pea and lemon soup
Barley salad*
Tomato and cress salad with creamy garlic dressing
Ginger sponge squares*

Day 5

½ grapefruit
Wholemeal baps with molasses
Herb tea or decaffeinated coffee

Jacket potato with mushrooms, peppers and walnuts
Fresh fruit

Leek and egg pie
Mixed green salad
Potato salad
Lemon sorbet

Day 6

Apple juice
Granola with fresh blackberries and soya or dairy milk
Herb tea or decaffeinated coffee

Hot corn-on-the-cob
Green salad with hazelnut dressing
French bread

Lentil and spinach curry*
Brown rice
Side dishes such as banana chunks, mango chutney, tomato salad
Indian sweets

Day 7

Mixed fruit juice
French toast with maple syrup
Herb tea or decaffeinated coffee

Creamy leek soup
Wholemeal baps
Salad garnish

Halloween party
Parsnip nut loaf*
Stuffed tomatoes*
Fennel and apple salad*
Lettuce dolmades*
Pasta salad
Green salad
Bread and crackers
Selection of cheeses
Pumpkin pie*

BORSCHT

3 medium sized raw beetroots, finely grated
1 onion, sliced
¼ small red cabbage, finely grated
850ml (1½ pints) vegetable stock
1 tablespoon lemon juice
1 teaspoon raw cane suger, or to taste
seasoning to taste
parsley and/or chives
sour cream, yogurt, tahini or concentrated soya milk – optional

Put the beetroot, onion, cabbage and vegetable stock into a saucepan. Bring to the boil, then lower the heat and simmer for 20 minutes. Do not cover.

Add lemon juice, sugar and seasoning as necessary.

Borscht can be blended to make a smooth soup, or served as it is. It can also be either chilled or eaten piping hot. Sprinkle with parsley and chives for extra flavour. Traditionally a swirl of sour cream or yogurt is added to each bowl just before serving borscht – but both tahini and soya milk make interesting alternatives.

LEEK AND ALMOND CRUMBLE

Filling:
4 large leeks, washed and sliced
2 large carrots, sliced
2 tablespoons vegetable oil
1 small onion, sliced
200ml (⅓ pint) vegetable stock
225g (8oz) ground almonds
115g (4oz) cooked peas
1 tablespoon wholemeal flour – optional
seasoning to taste
Topping:
2 tablespoons vegetable oil
115g (4oz) rolled oats
55g (2oz) almonds, coarsely chopped
seasoning to taste
½–1 teaspoon dried sage or thyme

Steam the leeks and carrots for 5 minutes to soften.

In a separate pan, heat the oil and cook the onion until tender but not coloured. Stir in most of the vegetable stock. Mix the almonds with the remaining stock and add to the pan. For a thicker sauce add the flour with the ground almonds. Add the peas, then the drained leeks and carrots. Stir so that the sauce is evenly distributed. Transfer the mixture to an ovenproof dish.

Make the topping by rubbing the oil into the oats and then stirring in the almonds, seasoning and herbs. Sprinkle this over the leek mixture, smooth the top with the back of a spoon. Bake at 350°F/190°C (Gas Mark 5) for 20 to 30 minutes, or until the crumble is crisp.

SPANISH QUICHE

Shortcrust pastry:
225g (8oz) wholemeal flour
pinch of salt
115g (4oz) margarine
approx. 2 tablespoons cold water
Filling:
1 small onion, thickly sliced
1 small green pepper, thickly sliced
2–3 tablespoons cooked peas
1 medium potato, cooked and cubed
3 small free-range eggs
200ml (1/3 pint) creamy milk
seasoning to taste
paprika
parsley

Make the pastry first. Sift together the flour and salt, then use fingertips to rub in the fat to make a mixture like crumbs. Add just enough water to make a soft but pliable dough. Wrap this in a polythene bag and chill in the fridge for 30 minutes.

Roll out the dough on a floured board then use to line a medium-sized flan dish (or flan ring on a baking sheet). Prick the base lightly and bake blind at 400°C/200°F (Gas Mark 6) for 10 minutes.

Scatter the onion, pepper, peas and potatoes across the base of the flan. Whisk together the eggs and milk, add seasoning and some paprika. Stir in coarsely chopped parsley. Pour the mixture over the vegetables. Bake at the same temperature for a further 20 to 30 minutes, or until the quiche is set.

CREAMED SWEETCORN PANCAKES

Pancakes:
2 free-range eggs or 55g (2oz) soya flour plus 1 teaspoon baking powder
pinch of salt
115g (4oz) wholemeal flour
285ml ($^1/_2$ pint) milk, milk and water, or water
vegetable oil for frying
Filling:
55g (2oz) margarine
1 large onion, sliced
1 large red pepper, sliced
340g (12oz) sweetcorn kernels*
55g (2oz) walnuts
seasoning to taste
140g (5oz) single cream or concentrated soya milk
2 tablespoons wholemeal breadcrumbs – optional
extra margarine – optional

Beat the eggs or combine the soya flour and baking powder, add salt, then the flour. Gradually stir in enough liquid to make a thin smooth cream. Beat lightly then set aside in a cool spot, preferably for 30 minutes.

To make the filling, melt the margarine, add the onion and pepper and cook gently to soften. Stir in the sweetcorn, walnuts and seasoning.

Beat the batter again. Heat a little oil in a thick-based frying pan, and pour in just 2 tablespoons of the batter, tilting the pan so that the batter spreads evenly. Cook until it begins to set, then toss or turn it with a spatula and cook the other side. Use the rest of the batter in the same way, keeping the pancakes hot (best on a plate over a saucepan of boiling water – cover the top too).

When the pancakes are ready, stir the cream or soya milk into the sweetcorn mixture and heat gently for just a minute. Divide the mixture between the pancakes and roll them up. You can serve them as they are, or arrange them side by side in a heatproof dish, top with breadcrumbs mixed with extra margarine, and put them under a hot grill for a few minutes.

*You can, of course, use frozen sweetcorn kernels, in which case cook and drain them first. Better still, cook fresh cobs and use a sharp knife to cut the kernels free.

MARROW RATATOUILLE WITH SMOKED TOFU

3 tablespoons vegetable oil
2 red peppers, sliced
2 onions, sliced
1–2 cloves of garlic, peeled and crushed
455g (1 lb) tomatoes, coarsely chopped
1 bay leaf
1 medium marrow, peeled, sliced and cut into cubes
seasoning to taste
fresh parsley
285g (10oz) smoked tofu, drained
extra vegetable oil

Heat the oil, gently fry the peppers, onions and garlic until soft. Stir in the tomatoes and bay leaf. Add the marrow cubes and cook for just 10 minutes or so, stirring often. Do not let the marrow become mushy. Remove the bay leaf. Add seasoning and parsley.

Meanwhile, cut the tofu into thin dominoes and fry these in oil until crisp and golden. Serve the ratatouille topped with the tofu.

BARLEY SALAD

115g (4oz) pot barley
850ml (1½ pints) vegetable stock
1 carrot, finely chopped
½ small cucumber, finely chopped
1 stick of celery, finely chopped
2 tablespoons raisins
55g (2oz) hazelnuts, preferably roasted
55g (2oz) peanuts, preferably roasted
1 tablespoon chopped fresh coriander or 1 teaspoon ground coriander
seasoning to taste

Cook the barley in the stock for 1 hour or until just tender, then drain off any excess liquid and rinse through with cold water. Drain again and place in a bowl.

Add all the other ingredients, mixing well. Chill briefly before serving.

GINGER SPONGE SQUARES

115g (4oz) margarine
115g (4oz) raw cane sugar
2 free-range eggs, lightly beaten
2 large tablespoons ginger conserve
55g (2oz) sultanas
½ teaspoon ground ginger, or to taste
140g (5oz) self-raising wholemeal flour

Cream together the margarine and sugar, stir in the eggs and mix well. Add the ginger conserve, sultanas, ground ginger and flour. The mixture should be thick and moist.

Grease a shallow cake tin, pour in the mixture, smooth the top. Bake at 375°F/190°C (Gas Mark 5) for 20 to 30 minutes. To check if sponge is cooked, press centre gently with your fingers. Remove from oven, cool slightly before cutting into squares. Transfer to a wire rack and leave to get cold.

LENTIL AND SPINACH CURRY

3 tablespoons vegetable oil
1 large onion, chopped
1 clove of garlic, peeled and crushed
1 teaspoon garam masala
1 teaspoon ground turmeric
½ teaspoon cumin
170g (6oz) split red lentils
200ml (⅓ pint) water
4 small potatoes, quartered
455g (1 lb) fresh spinach, washed and shredded
115g (4oz) creamed coconut, grated
85g (3oz) salted peanuts

Heat the oil and gently fry the onion and garlic for 5 minutes. Stir in the spices and fry for 5 minutes more (you can use made-up curry powder if you prefer, though the flavour won't be as rich). Add the lentils and water and bring to the boil, simmer for 10 minutes, add the potatoes. Continue cooking for 10 minutes more, or until the potatoes and lentils are tender.

Add the spinach to the pan and cook just long enough for it to soften. Check the liquid and add more if necessary, though don't make it too wet. Stir in the coconut so that it melts. Sprinkle the curry with peanuts just before serving it.

PARSNIP NUT LOAF

225g (8oz) mixed nuts, ground
225g (8oz) wholemeal breadcrumbs
2 tablespoons vegetable oil
1 medium onion, finely chopped
1 large parsnip, peeled and cubed
2 free-range eggs, lightly beaten
good pinch ground nutmeg
½ teaspoon dried marjoram
½ teaspoon dried thyme
seasoning to taste
parsley sprigs

Combine the nuts and breadcrumbs. Heat the oil and lightly fry the onion, then mix with the first ingredients. Steam the parsnip until soft enough to mash to a smooth purée, drain well, add to the mixture. Stir in the eggs, nutmeg, herbs and seasoning. The result should be a fairly firm mixture so you may need to add more crumbs and/or nuts or – if it is too stiff – a drop of water or vegetable stock.

Shape the mixture into a roll about 6″ in length, and place it on a well greased baking tray. Bake at 350°F/180°C (Gas Mark 4) for 30 minutes or until cooked. Cool, slice, decorate with parsley.

STUFFED TOMATOES

12 firm medium-sized tomatoes
225g (8oz) tofu, drained
55g (2oz) sunflower seeds, lightly roasted
soy sauce
1 tablespoon finely chopped basil or 1 teaspoon dried basil
seasoning to taste

Carefully slice the top off each tomato, scoop out the seeds with a spoon, stand the tomatoes upside down to drain.

Mash the tofu with the tomato innards plus sunflower seeds, soy sauce, basil and seasoning. Stuff some of the mixture back into each of the tomato shells, piling it high if necessary. Chill before serving.

FENNEL AND APPLE SALAD

2 large apples, coarsely grated
1 medium fennel bulb, coarsely grated
55g (2oz) walnut pieces – optional
French yogurt dressing:
140ml (¼ pint) plain yogurt
1 tablespoon vegetable oil
1 tablespoon white wine vinegar or lemon juice
seasoning to taste

Put the apples and fennel into a bowl. Mix the ingredients for the dressing thoroughly and pour them over the apple and fennel. Toss lightly, chill before serving. Sprinkle with walnuts if using them. A few of the fennel leaves make an attractive garnish.

LETTUCE DOLMADES

12 large lettuce leaves*
30g (1oz) margarine
3 spring onions or a small piece of sweet onion
6 mushrooms, chopped
55g (2oz) currants
55g (2oz) pine nuts
140g (5oz) brown rice, cooked
1 good teaspoon mixed spice
fresh mint and parsley, chopped
seasoning to taste
285ml (½ pint) vegetable stock

Cut off any hard stumps, then drop the leaves into a large pan of boiling water and cook for literally a few minutes to soften. Refresh them with cold water and pat dry.

Melt the margarine and lightly fry the onions and mushrooms. Stir in the currants, pine nuts, rice, spice, herbs and seasoning. Taste and adjust flavour if necessary.

Divide the mixture between the leaves, placing a spoonful at one end, folding the sides and then rolling it up to make a small parcel.

Arrange these close together in an overproof dish. Pour on the stock, cover the dish and bake at 350°F/180°C (Gas Mark 4) for about 20 minutes or until the leaves are tender. Lift out the dolmades one by one, drain them, serve either hot or cold. For a buffet party they are best served as they are, but at other times you could try them with a rich tomato sauce.

*Dolmades are actually stuffed vine leaves - if you want to do it the traditional way, look out in speciality shops for the right leaves. Otherwise you can use cos lettuce, Chinese leaves, or even cabbage. As these vary enormously in texture, adjust the cooking time accordingly.

PUMPKIN PIE

Shortcrust pastry: as for SPANISH QUICHE (above)
Filling:
455g (1 lb) pumpkin, peeled and de-seeded
½ teaspoon cinnamon
½ teaspoon ginger
½ teaspoon nutmeg
¼ teaspoon ground cloves
1–2 tablespoons honey or raw cane sugar
285ml (½ pint) creamy dairy or soya milk
1 tablespoon finely grated orange peel
raisins and/or walnuts – optional
whipped cream to serve – optional

Make up the pastry, roll out and line a flan ring that is resting on a baking tray. Bake blind at 400°F/200°C (Gas Mark 6) for 10 minutes.

Meanwhile, cut the pumpkin into cubes and steam until tender. Drain well, then mash to a purée. Mix this with the spices, sweetening and milk. Add the orange peel. You can also add raisins and nuts, if liked. Pour the mixture into the pastry base and return at once to the oven. Lower the heat to 350°F/180°C (Gas Mark 4) and cook for about 40 minutes, or until the filling is set. Serve warm or cold, cut into wedges. Nice with a dollop of whipped cream.

This pie is fairly soft in texture. If you prefer a firmer filling, either add 1 or 2 eggs, or use 1 tablespoon agar agar to set the pumpkin.

Winter

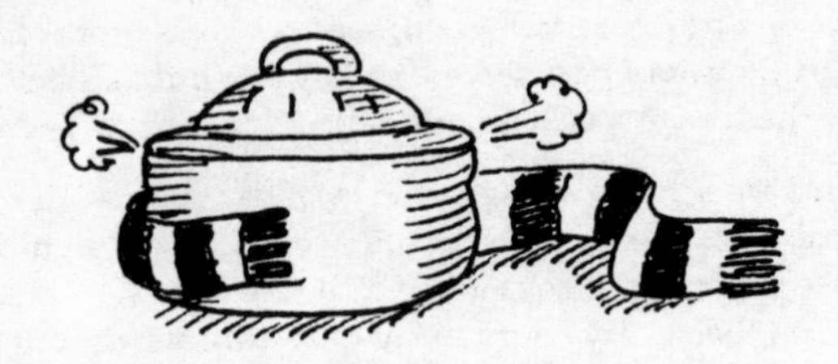

BREAKFAST	LUNCH	DINNER
Day 1		
Grapefruit juice Scrambled tofu on toast* Herb tea or decaffeinated coffee	Winter vegetable hot pot with butter beans Wholemeal bread Handful of fresh dates	Mushroom and chive soufflé omelette* French fried potatoes Brussels sprouts Pineapple slices
Day 2		
Mixed fruit juice Muffin with honey or marmalade Herb tea or decaffeinated coffee	Shepherd's pie with soya meat Endive and apple salad Wholemeal biscuits	Avocado vinaigrette Cheese fondue Wholemeal bread cubes and raw vegetables to dip Citrus fruit salad with ginger
Day 3		
½ grapefruit Granola with soya or dairy milk Herb tea or decaffeinated coffee	Celery and stilton soup* Vegetable pasty Carton of yogurt with honey	Moussaka with walnuts* Roast potatoes Leek salad Tofu cheesecake

Day 4

Pineapple and coconut drink
Oat bran cereal with soya or dairy milk
Herb tea or decaffeinated coffee

Wholemeal sandwiches with hummus and cucumber slices
Fresh fruit

Tagliatelle with pesto sauce*
Chicory salad
Dried pear mousse

Day 5

Orange juice with lemon
Granola with soya or dairy milk
Herb tea or decaffeinated coffee

Nut butter and watercress sandwiches
Tomato salad
Dried fruit and nut bar

Baked avocado*
Jacket potato
Red cabbage salad
Baked apple with cashew cream

Day 6

Apricot juice
Shredded Wheat with sultanas and soya or dairy milk
Herb tea or decaffeinated coffee

Parsnip ramekins
Herb muffins
Celery, apple and walnut salad
Dried fruit bar

Chili tempura with dips*
Watercress and endive salad
Hot bulgar
Fresh fruit salad with rosewater

Day 7

Orange juice
Tropical muesli* with soya or dairy milk
Herb tea or decaffeinated coffee

Christmas lunch
Melon surprise*
Brussels sprouts and hazelnut bake*
Carrot sauce*
Jacket potatoes
Chicory and red pepper salad
Mincemeat strudel*
Cream or coconut cream

Vegetarian Scotch eggs
Tomato and cucumber salad
Wholemeal bread
Fresh fruit

SCRAMBLED TOFU ON TOAST (for one)

1 tablespoon vegetable oil
140g (5oz) tofu, drained and mashed
good pinch of turmeric
soy sauce
garlic salt
fresh ground pepper
2 slices wholemeal bread

Heat the oil and add the tofu, stirring it constantly. Sprinkle with turmeric, soy sauce, salt and pepper to flavour.

Lightly toast the bread (add butter or margarine if liked), pile on the scrambled tofu and eat whilst hot.

MUSHROOM AND CHIVE SOUFFLÉ OMELETTE

6 free-range eggs
approx. 55g (2oz) margarine
115g (4oz) mushrooms, cleaned and sliced
chives
seasoning to taste

Separate the eggs and whisk the whites until stiff.

Using a large pan, melt the margarine and gently cook the mushrooms, turning them so that they colour evenly.

Beat the egg yolks with a little water, plus the chives and seasoning. Carefully stir in the whites. Pour the mixture into the pan (adding more fat first if necessary). Cook the mixture gently until it sets underneath. Then put it under a grill to cook on top. Do not fold to serve, but cut into thick wedges instead.

CELERY AND STILTON SOUP

2 tablespoons vegetable oil
1 medium head of celery, thinly sliced
1 medium onion, thinly sliced
30g (1oz) wholemeal flour
a good 850ml (1½ pints) vegetable stock
55g (2oz) stilton (or other blue cheese), crumbled
freshly ground black pepper
parsley and croûtons

Heat the oil and cook the celery and onion to soften. Stir in the flour and cook a minute more, then add the vegetable stock. Bring to the boil, cover the pan and simmer for about 20 minutes. If you like a smoother soup, liquidise it at this stage.

Gradually whisk in the cheese, making sure the soup does not boil. Check flavour and adjust if necessary. Add freshly ground black pepper to taste. Serve very hot with plenty of parsley and wholemeal croûtons.

MOUSSAKA WITH WALNUTS

1 large aubergine
approx. 4 tablespoons vegetable oil
1 large onion, sliced
2 medium courgettes, chopped
4 tomatoes, peeled and chopped
3 tablespoons red wine – optional
1 teaspoon mixed herbs
85g (3oz) walnuts, coarsely ground
30g (1oz) wholemeal breadcrumbs
seasoning to taste
30g (1oz) wholemeal flour
285ml (½ pint) dairy or soya milk
parsley to garnish

Slice the aubergine, lay on a plate and sprinke with salt. After 30 minutes, wash the slices in fresh water and pat dry.

Heat half the oil and cook the aubergine slices on both sides until tender, then set aside to drain. Add another tablespoon of oil to the pan and cook the onion for 5 minutes. Stir in the courgettes and continue cooking. After a few minutes, add the tomatoes, wine and herbs and cook gently until a sauce forms. Stir in the nuts and crumbs, add flavouring. The mixture should be thick and moist – add water, oil or some tomato purée if it seems too dry.

Make a white sauce with the remaining tablespoon of oil, flour and milk, seasoning it well.

Lightly grease a small ovenproof dish. Put half the aubergine in the bottom, cover with half the nut mix and half the white sauce. Repeat this to use the remaining ingredients. Bake at 350°F/180°C (Gas Mark 4) for about 30 minutes. Garnish with parsley.

TAGLIATELLE WITH PESTO SAUCE

28g (10oz) tagliatelle, preferably wholemeal
Parmesan cheese to serve
Pesto sauce:
1–2 cloves of garlic, peeled and crushed
1–2 tablespoons fresh basil leaves
85g (3oz) Parmesan cheese, grated
85g (3oz) pine nuts
1 tablespoon lemon juice
approx. 140ml (1/4 pint) olive oil
seasoning to taste

Cook the pasta according to instructions. This depends on whether it is fresh or dried; either way it will not take much more than 10 minutes to soften.

The sauce can be made in advance and kept until needed. Use a mortar and pestle to grind all the dry ingredients, mix in the lemon juice, then slowly add the oil, drop by drop, making sure it is well blended before adding more. The final mixture should be the consistency of a thin cream. You can make it in a liquidiser if you prefer, stirring in the cheese by hand at the end.

Whilst draining the pasta, put one or two tablespoons of pesto sauce per person into the pan, and heat gently for literally a minute or two. Stir into the pasta and serve at once. You can sprinkle it with extra cheese if liked, and add more pepper.

Pesto sauce is a very special sauce that relies for its subtle flavour on *fresh* basil. If you cannot get fresh leaves, it would be better to buy one of the excellent ready-made sauces now available, including a vegan version.

BAKED AVOCADO

4 large avocados, ripe but still firm
lemon juice
2 slices wholemeal bread, made into crumbs
55g (2oz) hazelnuts, roasted and coarsely chopped
4 tomatoes, chopped
1 stick of celery, chopped
½ teaspoon dried mixed herbs
seasoning to taste
vegetable stock or water, or 1 egg
85g (3oz) cheddar cheese, grated – optional
30g (1oz) margarine – optional

Cut the avocados in half, remove the stones. If preferred you can also cut away the skin. Brush the surface with lemon juice.

In a bowl mix together the breadcrumbs, hazelnuts, tomatoes, celery, herbs, seasoning, and enough liquid or egg to bind.

Arrange the avocado halves in an overproof dish and divide the filling between them. If liked, top with grated cheese or knobs of margarine.

Bake at 400°F/200°C (Gas Mark 6) for 20 minutes. Serve hot.

CHILI TEMPURA WITH DIPS

Batter:
115g (4oz) self raising wholemeal flour
½ teaspoon chili powder
1 free-range egg
200ml (⅓ pint) iced water
1 tablespoon vegetable oil
Vegetables:
1 large parsnip, peeled and cubed
1 large carrot, peeled and cubed
1 medium onion, peeled and cut into rings
1 stick of celery, cut into segments
12 button mushrooms
1 yellow pepper, cubed
wholemeal flour for coating
vegetable oil for deep frying

Sift together the flour and chili powder. Whisk in the egg and then the water and oil to make a batter that is thick and smooth.

Prepare the vegetables. Heat the oil. Dust the vegetables with flour, then dip them into the batter and drop them into the oil a few at a time. They should change colour in about 3 minutes. Drain them on paper towels and keep them warm whilst cooking the rest in the same way.

Dips to serve with chili tempura vegetables are up to you – a selection is a good idea. Try mixing sour cream with a little yogurt and add fresh herbs. Or mash up some avocados with lemon juice and mayonnaise or cream. Tofu and tahini make an excellent dip too. Use your imagination.

TROPICAL MUESLI

1.15 kilos (2 lbs) mixed cereal grain
115g (4oz) flaked coconut, roasted
115g (4oz) dried banana chips
115g (4oz) candied or dried pineapple
115g (4oz) dried mangoes, chopped
55g (2oz) raw cane sugar
2–3 teaspoons mixed spice
115g (4oz) Brazil nuts, coarsely chopped

Combine all the ingredients and store in a large jar. Use as needed. Good with soya or dairy milk, yogurt, or diluted fruit juices such as orange. Soaking overnight makes it creamy.

MELON SURPRISE

2 small honeydew melons
2 tablespoons lemon juice
2 tablespoons chopped stem ginger
port or juice from preserved ginger
55g (2oz) walnut pieces, chopped
24 green grapes

Halve the melons, use a spoon to scoop out the seeds. Stand them upside down to drain.

Mix the lemon juice with the stem ginger, plus enough port or juice to moisten well, and the walnut pieces and grapes. Fill the melon halves with this mixture. Chill well before serving, adding a drop more port or juice if liked.

BRUSSELS SPROUTS AND HAZELNUT BAKE

455g (1 lb) Brussels sprouts, washed and trimmed
2 carrots, peeled and coarsely chopped
4 slices wholemeal bread, made into crumbs
140ml (1/4 pint) milk
115g (4oz) hazelnuts, coarsely ground
2 free-range eggs
170g (6oz) cheddar cheese, grated
seasoning to taste
good pinch ground nutmeg
extra hazelnuts for topping, coarsely chopped – optional

Steam the sprouts and carrots until tender, then drain well and mash.

Soak the bread in the milk for 10 minutes. Add the sprouts and carrots together with the nuts. Separate the eggs and stir the yolks into the mixture. Add the grated cheese, seasoning and nutmeg. Whisk the egg whites until stiff, then use a metal spoon to fold them into the vegetables.

Grease a small ovenproof dish or loaf tin and spoon in the mixture, smoothing the top. Bake at 350°F/180°C (Gas Mark 4) for about 45 minutes, or until set. If using hazelnuts for topping, sprinkle them over the loaf after 30 minutes.

Remove carefully from the tin and serve cut in slices, with carrot sauce (see next recipe).

CARROT SAUCE

425ml (3/4 pint) vegetable stock
285g (10oz) carrots, peeled and chopped
1 large onion, peeled and chopped
seasoning to taste
thyme, parsley and chives
tahini – optional

Combine all the ingredients in a small saucepan and cook for about 10 minutes, or until the carrot is soft. Liquidise to make a thick, smooth sauce. Adjust flavouring, add more herbs as necessary. Heat through gently and serve hot. A spoonful or two of tahini stirred in at the last moment makes the sauce creamier.

MINCEMEAT STRUDEL

225g (8oz) filo pastry
approx. 115g (4oz) margarine or butter, melted
455g (1 lb) vegetarian mincemeat
a little apple juice or brandy
raw cane icing sugar – optional

If the pastry is frozen, leave it to defrost. Separate the layers carefully and lay them out flat. Cover with a tea towel to prevent them drying.

Grease a shallow baking tin. Cover the base with a single layer of the pastry and use a pastry brush to dab it lightly with fat. Use half the sheets in this way, laying them one on top of the other, and making sure each one is brushed right to the edges with fat.

Cover with a thick layer of mincemeat, adding a drop of apple juice or brandy to make it more moist. Then lay the rest of the pastry on top, one layer at a time, brushing fat over each one. The top layer will need extra fat to keep it from buckling.

Use a sharp knife to mark the strudel into diamonds.

Bake at 375°F/190°C (Gas Mark 5) for about 20 minutes, or until crisp and golden. Remove from the oven and dust the top with icing sugar (if you can't find this in the shops, make your own by powdering raw cane sugar in a grinder). Leave to cool slightly before cutting through. Serve warm or cold.

Reference Sources

The Allergy Problem, Vicky Rippere, Thorsons, 1983.
This Food Business, New Statesmen and Society, 1989.
The Reduction Factor, Weight Watchers, 1989.
The Food Scandal, C. Walker & G. Cannon, Century Publishing, 1985.
Dieting Makes You Fat, G. Cannon & H. Einzig, Century Publishing, 1983.